Support for Family and Friends

Caring for someone with a long-term illness

John Costello

D0549835

Manchester University Press

Manchester and New York

distributed in the United States exclusively by Palgrave Macmillan

Published by Manchester University Press
Oxford Road, Manchester M13 9NR, UK
and Room 400, 175 Fifth Avenue, New York, NY 10010, USA
www.manchesteruniversitypress.co.uk

Distributed in the United States exclusively by
Palgrave Macmillan, 175 Fifth Avenue, New York,
NY 10010, USA

Distributed in Canada exclusively by
UBC Press, University of British Columbia, 2029 West Mall,
Vancouver, BC, Canada V6T 1Z2

British Library Cataloguing-in-Publication Data
A catalogue record for this book is available from the British Library

Library of Congress Cataloging-in-Publication Data applied for

ISBN 978 0 7190 7805 7   *hardback*
     978 0 7190 7806 4   *paperback*

First published 2009

18 17 16 15 14 13 12 11 10 09   10 9 8 7 6 5 4 3 2 1

The publisher has no responsibility for the persistance or accuracy of URLs for external or any third-party internet websites referred to in this book, and does not guarantee that any content on such websites is, or will remain, accurate or appropriate.

Note: the advice and information included in this book is published in good faith. However, both the author and the publisher assume no responsibility or liability for any injury, loss or expense incurred as a result of relying on the information stated. Please check with the relevant authorities regarding any changes in legislation since publication.

Typeset in Stone Serif with Stone display
by Koinonia, Manchester
Printed in Great Britain
by the MPG Books Group

Contents

Introduction

There are estimated to be over 6 million carers in the UK – an eighth of the population – combining their caring role with paid employment. It has been calculated that carers currently save the economy £57 billion annually in care costs. This is the equivalent of a second NHS! Three million of these 6 million carers in the UK juggle work with their role as carer. Long-term illness, often referred to as chronic illness, is now the main reason why people seek health care in the Western world.

This book is designed for those people who have made a conscious decision to care for and offer support to the millions of people in the UK with a long-term illness. It discusses the experience of being a carer for a person with a long-term illness. It is not about specific diseases. Long-term illness is often unpredictable and complex and in itself is not amenable to simple discussion about any one aspect of the disease. It is having a condition where pathological changes occur in the body that are irreversible, permanent or leave residual disability. The condition may be characterized by periods of recurrence and remission, such as with multiple sclerosis (MS). People with long-term illness generally require extended periods of care, supervision and observation. Having a long-term illness does not necessarily mean an immediate and sustained need for nursing care. 'Long-term illness' can include conditions such as diabetes, renal disease, some cancers, heart disease, cerebral palsy, muscular dystrophy, arthritis and many neurological diseases, such as MS, motor neurone disease (MND) and Parkinson's disease. The list is not comprehensive and, like many of these illnesses, people experience prolonged periods where the symptoms are active, as well as times when the illness appears to lie dormant. Having a long-term condition does not always mean being ill. Moreover, it is a state of being which describes the whole experience of the person who lives with the disease. What is clear is that for many people there is no cure for their condition. Despite the many advances in medical science, for those with long-term conditions medical intervention is focused on controlling and alleviating their symptoms but offers no cure. For many their condition means never returning to a 'normal state'; most people live with their condition rather than die from it. In the past, many people would not have lived long enough to reach the advanced stages of their illness that many do today. This is largely due to advances in medical science, as well as progress in the standard of medical and nursing care.

What is long-term illness?

In contemporary society, 'long-term illness' has become an ambiguous term, with people suffering from a wide range of symptoms, some of which are rarely fully diagnosed. It has been estimated that 60 per cent of people in England report a chronic health problem that is both physical and psychological in origin. This includes diabetes mellitus (1.3 million, with another 1 million who may be undiagnosed).

Long-term illnesses are often prolonged, do not resolve spontaneously and are rarely cured completely. In England, 8.8 million people report having a long-term illness that *severely limits their day-to-day ability to cope*. The persistence of symptoms over time, with or without asymptomatic (without symptoms) periods, suggests chronicity, especially when there is no specific cure. I recently discovered that my GP practice classifies me as *a chronic or long-term illness sufferer,* as I have now had asthma for 16 years. The fact that few people who know me realize I have asthma is immaterial, as is the fact that it is well controlled and I require little medication. My GP is inclined to think that, since I have not been cured, then *my asthma* is long-term in nature. I attend an annual asthma check and receive good reports confirming that it is well controlled. My illness allows me to qualify for a free flu jab every year. However, the type of long-term illness I focus on in this book is the type that requires someone to assist the person with the condition – albeit not all the time, as there may be times when a person with cancer (which may be considered a long-term condition for many people) will be fully independent. There may also be other times when a person with Alzheimer's disease who is being cared for at home will require 24-hour care.

The term 'long-term illness' may be more accurately described as illness that does not quickly or easily become cured, and by definition refers to illnesses that people experience for the rest of their lives. This book focuses on the role played by the carer in supporting the person with a long-term condition and I hope that it is helpful to both parties, despite the emphasis being placed on lay care providers as opposed to professional care providers. As a nurse and lecturer in health-related topics, I have been interested in the social experience of illness for many years – an experience that is shaped by the disease process, the character of the patient (I dislike the word sufferer or victim) and the context in which care takes place. I think it important to stress at this point that, despite my nursing background, I acknowledge that for many people institutional care (although important) is not their preferred place of care, but in some cases it is essential and important. This book focuses on the care provided in community settings, specifically in the home. My relatively brief experience as a carer for my father with cancer taught me a lot about the needs of people with debilitating illness. I also learned how difficult it was to become an effective carer! I assumed many years ago that my nursing background would prepare me for the role of carer but in reality it was a shock to have to change from being a nurse, having hospital resources available all the time, to 'making do' with the everyday things in a home environment. Caring as a professional and as a layperson are different experiences. This book is for all the people who care for others with a condition that prevents them from doing the things that many of us take for granted. It is written to help carers have good experiences, so that the experience of being a carer can become fulfilling and, when reflected upon, can bring satisfaction to both the carer and the cared for.

About this book

The book consists of seven chapters, each with a specific focus. Chapter 1 addresses the personal attributes of the carer. It considers the role and responsibilities of the carer and considers some of the things that influence how we care and what type of carer we will become. I include a short section on carer assessment, which is the formal assessment made by social workers. The chapter also considers patient and carer attitudes, as well as examining how the media often portray people as battling certain diseases, such as cancer. I felt that it was important to look at what influences the way we care, so I have discussed what the academic literature says about being a carer. This is the only chapter where I look at the wider evidence and research in detail; I think it is important to consider the carer's image and people's expectations of carers. I also include a section on the relationship that carers develop with other health and social care professionals.

Chapter 2 looks more closely at practical issues, taking a 'how' and 'what-to-do' approach to focusing on the practical issues that can occur when caring for someone with a long-term illness. The chapter examines the most common problems using what many health care professionals call an Activities of Daily Living approach (ADL).

Chapter 3 addresses the experience of pain and discomfort, focusing on how to assess and manage pain.

Chapter 4 focuses on those everyday things we do in life that we take for granted and are known professionally as Activities of Daily Living (ADL). In particular, it looks at a particular aspect of care described by many as the British disease – the so-called obsession with bowel and bladder problems.

Chapter 5 looks at psychological care. It focuses on the use of effective interpersonal skills to enable the patient to express their concerns and receive empathic responses from the carer that will help to meet the patient's psychological needs. The chapter uses case-study evidence to illustrate how important it is that carers are able to listen to the patient, identify their emotional needs and make appropriate responses. In particular the chapter considers the growing problem of patients with a range of neurological problems, specifically confusion.

Chapter 6 focuses on the management of dying, which is included because it is the reality of caring for people with a life-threatening illness; the outcome of their experience of the illness is inevitable death. Not to discuss this sad but important aspect of human experience is to avoid an important part of being a carer. The chapter considers the many sensitive issues involved when the patient's illness has progressed to the stage where they require palliative care and may be facing impending death. It will consider three main areas: advancing illness and decision making about the future; the need for palliative/terminal care; and the practical issues involved in making a living will and what to do as death approaches.

Chapter 7 considers the well-being of the carer as a valued part of the care provided to the person with a long-term illness. The aim of this chapter is to identify and describe sources of help for carers and how to access them, but at the same time it considers the situation where carers hold down paid employment while also being a carer. The chapter identifies sources of support from support groups and self-help strategies for enabling the carer to develop and maintain their own well-being. The chapter also considers some of the financial and practical sources of help for the patient, who may be eligible for allowances and benefits – such as attendance allowance –

that can be used to help them to pay for care and support.

For clarity I refer to people being cared for as patients, partly because it is a term that encapsulates a wide range of meanings, but also because it is accurate for many – albeit, I appreciate, not applicable to all. The book focuses on adults but also contains references that teenagers and other youngsters may find useful. To enable readers to learn more about different terms used throughout the book (as if you need to know!) and to improve clarity, I have included a glossary of terms, as well as a list of useful contacts and helpful organizations. The book is intended as a resource to add to the knowledge that carers quickly gain on their illness journey. I hope it helps to make this journey a more satisfying and enlightening one, for the carer as well as those for whom they care.

1

On becoming a carer

This chapter has two purposes: to consider what we mean by long-term illness and to look at the role of the lay carer for someone with a long-term illness. It begins by looking closely at what we call long term and at the differences and similarities between acute illness and chronic or long-term illness. The second part of the chapter considers what constitutes caring and looks at the role of the carer for someone with a long-term illness, including a discussion of what the role involves and the qualities of the carer. The chapter explains the importance of both physical and psychological care, as well as examining how attitude makes a difference to the understanding of the illness and the image of the carer. I also discuss the importance of carers having the ability to assess the patient's emotional state (emotional IQ), and use case studies of people with long-term illness and their carers.

What do we mean by long-term illness?

The experience of illness has changed dramatically in the last hundred years. Traditionally, illness and disease at the turn of the last century was almost always of a relatively short duration and was invariably due to infection. Disease such as cholera, typhoid fever and tuberculosis (consumption) affected millions of the labouring classes and others. Consumption often resulted in death after 6 to 12 weeks, the afflicted took to their death beds and passed away, with weight loss and fever the dominant features of their short illness. In modern times, illness is often defined as a 'period of disease' or sickness is described as being of 'sudden onset'. Acute episodes of illness can be physical or psychological and render the person temporarily unable to perform their normal day-to-day activities. This can include a chest infection, a migraine, a period of depression or food poisoning. The physical requirements of long-term care can be the same as an acute episode, although they tend to be classified as being of longer duration, with periods where the person is symptom-free (remission periods), and at the same time acute episodes can occur. A person can have a condition called chronic obstructive pulmonary disease (COPD, traditionally known as chronic bronchitis) but also have acute episodes of infection. In this case they have a long-standing condition with shorter flare-ups due to a chest infection. People with arthritis (rheumatoid and osteoarthritis) can also have acute periods when they often feel much worse. The more long-term illnesses such as MND, MS and Parkinson's disease, all of which are classified as long-term, also include periods when the person feels much worse than at other times. A person with depression that continues for a long time, over many years, may be regarded as having chronic depression, simply because it does not relinquish despite medication and various therapies. Long-term care can include a wide range of diseases, the origins of which can be physical, such as cancer, or psychological illness, such as schizophrenia, Alzheimer's disease or depression.

What is caring?

The carer role is a very responsible one that people take very seriously. To care for another person is an important task as well as a very privileged position to be in. For some professional caregivers, caring is an everyday activity, which some may take for granted because it is a routine work-related activity. It was only when my wife and I accepted the task of caring for my father that I began to appreciate that, when you take on the unpaid carer's role outside of your normal job, it is very different and difficult (see Costello 1990, 2004).

Caring for someone with a long-term illness is a special activity. The caregiver has to make many decisions about what it means to them, what they are going to do and how they intend to do it. Being a carer means giving of yourself, making a commitment to provide time, energy and, according to Griffin (1981), love for another person. This other person does not have to be a relative or friend, but someone who you care about and decide to care for. The love is said to be a moderated kind of love, based on the assumption that to provide the best kind of care involves not only doing things for that person but also caring for them by extending personal human skills such as kindness, empathy and compassion. Caring involves commitment to another, which involves practical commitments to being there, giving time and spending that time to enable the person to feel better. People affected by a different disease (which may include long-term disease) not only require physical care but psychological care also. Carers are often capable of meeting and fulfilling the physical requirements of care, which can include positioning a person in bed, administering medication, helping them to eat and drink or get to the toilet. In fact, after a while many carers may begin to wonder how their role differs from that of professional nurses in hospitals. Providing high-quality physical care is important and very necessary. Those dependent on others to get out of bed appreciate others who turn up on time and have warm hands and gentle handling techniques. Without someone 'doing' and 'seeing to', the many essential activities of daily living (ADL – of which more later), many dependent people with long-term illness would deteriorate, become unhappy, more dependent and in some cases die sooner. It is important that carers provide high-quality practical care, as this has a direct bearing on the person's well-being. Changing an indwelling urinary catheter bag seems like an easy task until you understand the cross-infection risks involved and the need to take universal precautions (see Chapter 4, 'Specific activities of daily living'). The challenge for many carers is to provide the more complex psychosocial aspects of care.

Psychological care

For some people with a long-term illness, having someone to carry out or help them with physical aspects of care is enough to keep them going and sufficient for their day-to-day care. This physical level of what some refer to as basic care often also involves a degree of psychological care, as no practical task is conducted in silence. Social services care providers are able to provide practical assistance to people with conditions ranging from strokes to Alzheimer's disease, often with very little time allocated to do this.

Providing psychological care can often take place at the same time as practical care and does not mean sitting face to face spending time in conversation (although this is often a very pleasant thing to do!). Care providers with little available time, such as social services caregivers, often give the people they visit the type of social and emotional support they require, while also having to carry out practical activities, such as assisting with washing and dressing. This is often not ideal and carers will often say, 'Oh, I wish I had more time to sit and talk to her, as she seems to be so lonely and in need of company.' Many people with long-term illness, particularly older people who live alone, require emotional support, not only because they are lonely but also because they are often frustrated by their condition. They find themselves becoming dependent and isolated, as they are unable to leave the house unaided. Their anxiety is often associated with uncertainty about the future and many experience a range of psychosocial difficulties, such as:

● dependency
● isolation
● fear of dying

- frustration
- depression
- fatigue*

*Fatigue is more than physical (see Chapter 7, 'Getting help and support'), and often involves the person feeling fed up and experiencing despair.

The qualities of a carer: caring as therapy

One of the major challenges of supporting a person with a long-term illness is to provide both physical and psychological care according to need. Nurses often refer to this as holistic care. This means taking into account that the person has a range of needs above and beyond the physical. In order to meet these needs, it is useful to go back and consider what Griffin (1981) considers to be the emotional aspects of caring. According to Griffin, the carer needs to consider that the relationship between the carer and the care provider can in itself be developed so that it has therapeutic value. By therapeutic I am referring to the ability of the relationship between the carer and care provider to provide support and healing – the carer, in becoming involved with the person, has the potential to do something therapeutic. That does not mean to say that all relationships in themselves are therapeutic; a person can have a gardener to take care of the garden or a cleaner to clean the house, but the relationship between the two does not involve therapy unless the potential for the care provider to develop their role with the other is borne in mind.

Gosia Brykczynska (1992) writes about caring as a dying art, pointing out that a carer can be competent but it does not make them a good carer. On the one hand caring may be seen as a natural state of being, but on the other it is a skilled art that requires education, training and moral integrity. However, the reader may ask: what is there to learn? The answer lies, perhaps, in learning to share oneself truly with others. What we need to learn about caring may be answered by another nurse (Roach 1985), who identified what has become known as the 'Five Cs of Caring'. These principles are not just for professional carers (although they were written for this audience), as they also have application for lay carers (such as the people who read this book), both of whom need to consider what is required to provide quality care to those we have decided to care for. The five Cs are:

- compassion
- competence
- confidence
- conscience
- commitment

The five principles relate to human qualities and are not unique to professional care providers. To have compassion is to have feelings for the other person. Compassion is said to be a prerequisite to becoming a carer. Compassion is more than pity and, despite finding yourself having to care, it is possible to have feelings for the person for whom you care. When my father was diagnosed as having bowel cancer, it quickly dawned on me that we would have to care for him in our home, as he lived alone and was dependent on others. My wife could not bear the thought of him dying in hospital. It was not a decision we took, but more an inevitability that occurred. For 15 months he lived with us and shared our lives, and eventually died in our front room (Costello 2004). When Roach (1985) discusses competence, she means the ability to have an enquiring mind and not to focus on doing tasks, but looking beyond what is required to develop a caring attitude. Confidence in caring is about being able to feel confident – an exuded form of confidence – but also about enabling the person being cared for to feel confident in you as a carer and to be able to trust you and what you do for them. In doing this, people make themselves vulnerable, as they *put themselves in your hands*. This is where the powerful notion of caring comes in, and the sometimes awesome responsibility begins to emerge. The carer also has to have a conscience or a sense of moral integrity, about not only what they do, but also when to decide that you require help. Roach (1985) points out that conscience is the sensitivity and informed sense of what is right and wrong, which acts like a compass, directing behaviour accordingly towards prescribed moral standards. Conscience is also highly personal and may involve taking certain risks and allowing the person being cared for to do what they truly want, within prescribed boundaries. This is considered in more detail in Chapter 6, where I discuss issues such as living wills. Finally, in terms of caring principles, others expect the carer to show commitment. This can be the most challenging aspect. Many of us are prepared to stand up and become the care provider when others would not, but fail to see the implications of the decision one year down the line, when things become difficult to sustain, the cared-for person is more dependent, their illness deteriorates, their disease progresses. It is at these points when we review our commitment and consider if we are still able and willing to carry on the care provider role (see Chapter 5, page 86).

The following case study may prove useful as an illustration of how lay carers can demonstrate some (if not all) the five Cs without necessarily having been educated and trained to a high level.

Case study: Amy

Amy was an 85-year-old lady with chronic arthritis, diagnosed at the age of 67. She lived alone in a small bungalow on the edge of a large council estate. Her condition had become worse in the last 5 years since the death of her husband Eric. She had one daughter who lived in Essex who visited every month. Amy was dependent on Social Service carers for daily help with getting up, dressing, washing and toileting. She was able to eat if the food was prepared in advance, and she could control her TV, read and listen to the radio during the day. Amy had three carers, who came daily. Her favourite was Kirsty because she was lively, chatty and Amy liked to hear about her young daughters (2 and 4). Kirsty was different to other carers: she seemed interested in Amy – conveyed through her tone of voice, touch and sense of warmth – which brought great comfort in the short 30 minutes Kirsty was there. Moreover, she seemed to like being with Amy, she did 'special things' for her, like fetching her favourite soap from the shop and telephoning her and getting the children to say 'Hello'. One day she even brought her two girls round for 10 minutes in the afternoon on her day off. Kirsty was different because, despite her age (26), she seemed to understand Amy's situation more than the others. Amy said she 'seemed to care about me as a person and not as the old cripple that I feel as if I am sometimes. Kirsty makes me laugh. The things she says, so uplifting, gives me a sense of confidence about myself.' More than anything she was always kind, considerate and thoughtful. Kirsty would invariably turn up on time and if not would phone and leave a voice-mail message over the speaker. Amy pointed out that it was not the reliability she appreciated; it was the joy of having a real live human being in her company, who seemed to like her for who she was rather than what she had become.

Being there

In the scenario, without knowing it, Kirsty was attending to Amy's emotional need to feel wanted and cared for. In various ways Kirsty demonstrated the principles of caring and was sincere in doing so. While it was her job to care, she seemed to do it effortlessly and with feeling. The practical aspects of care were always carried out (maybe not always 100 per cent efficiently), but Amy's need for comfort and perhaps to feel accepted were met through a caring medium generated by the care provider who, Griffin (1981) would say, 'developed a relationship based on a form of love for the other person'. Carers who have the responsibility of moving and handling others can convey their feelings in the way they move people. Older people in hospital who are often moved by nurses, come to recognize nurses who are 'heavy-handed' or careless in the way they touch people. Sensitivity comes from within the carer. Ellen Newton, in her book *This Bed my Center* (1988), discusses the personalities of different carers she encountered in her journey from dependency to independency. She recognized that in institutions for older people some carers gave the most valuable commodity time, more readily than others. These same people were able to convey warmth and compassion towards the residents and, by recognizing their individuality, made them feel like people.

Becoming a carer: formal assessment

In order to become a formally acknowledged and registered carer, all carers need to undergo a basic assessment of their duties and role, which is conducted by staff from the local Social Services department. The assessment is a process conducted by social workers at the place where you provide care and involves talking to you and the patient. Often it takes one visit, although it could involve two or three separate visits. The purpose of the assessment is to find out what you are expected to do as a carer, whether you are able to do this and what (if any) support you require. The assessment considers the following areas:

- the patient's problems, diagnosis and medical needs
- the suitability of the care environment
- daily routine, aspects of the carer's role
- what difficulties exist for carer and patient
- degree of support required (carer and patient)
- specialist advice or help required to become a carer.

The key thing to consider regarding the assessment is that it is a helping process that identifies areas of need and support, not a test or examination of your ability. It can often be combined with a community care assessment that is focused on the patient, and conducted at the same time, if the patient is eligible. Before the visit, it is useful to make a list of your needs including need for rest, leisure, outside interests and areas where you require more knowledge, skill or specialist advice.

Bear in mind that the assessment is to help you become a more effective carer. Therefore it is worth making a pre-assessment list of your needs for practical advice as well as information, financial advice, work status, employment issues (if part-time worker) and support to help you if you have a family or other work or social commitments. Remember also that it is always useful to involve the person you are caring for in arranging a carer assessment, as they play a big part and can be helpful in terms of highlighting long-term needs and the ability to plan for the future.

The qualities of a carer

What was it about Kirsty and what she did for Amy that made Amy feel that she was meeting her needs? Could it have been the way she did things, rather than the outcome of her efforts? Often when we feel low in mood or generally fed up, talking to someone who understands is helpful. Many writers have discussed this so-called *talking therapy* over the years in terms of people emotionally engaging with each other – in other words, moving beyond the words and reaching out to connect with the speaker's feelings. Perhaps this is what Kirsty was trying to do, and she seemed to be doing it well! It could be said that Kirsty had what is called a high *emotional IQ* – the ability for one person to engage with others enough to perceive their emotional state (and sometimes the reason for it). A carer who is able to identify the patient's emotional needs, and uses this understanding to drive their thinking and behaviour, is able to manage the relationship to good effect. We often talk about intelligence as a desirable asset to the personality, but having the ability to assess what emotions are being raised by someone is like being able to decode a message. Often there is a difference between listening to what others say and under-standing the emotions being expressed. Read Glynnis's case study and try to distinguish the facts from the subjective comment.

Case study: Glynnis

Glynnis (75) lives alone and is being treated with steroids for her arthritis. She is able to get to the toilet with assistance but is dependent on carers (who visit twice a day) and her neighbour (for shopping). The health visitor comes round to do a three-monthly visit to assess her general state of health. Glynnis points out that she often feels tired and fed up. Her neighbour (Hilda) comes in every day and does some shopping, but cannot stay long as she cares for her elderly infirm husband. Glynnis enjoys the television but wakes early every day, and it takes her two hours to get up and sit in the chair, due to joint pain. She says she may as well be dead, as some days she feels so stiff she cannot move until she has taken her medication. The evenings are the worst, she says, since no one comes round after 6.00pm.

Glynnis is lonely. She craves company and someone to talk to and spend time with. She appears to have come to terms with her illness and the dependency it places on her, although her greatest need is for physical company, which seems to be rationed.

The carer's image

Caring for a person with a long-term illness can be rewarding, challenging and very, very daunting. For some, being praised all the time and thought of as a Florence Nightingale character can be hard to bear. Lay carers experience a range of different positive and negative self-images, feeling self-righteous, a martyr, overwhelmed, unsupported, intimidated and out of their depth. Why do carers experience these emotions and how does it help shape their self-image?

It is important to consider that the carer's role in helping to manage a person with long-term illness is very challenging. Irrespective of the type of illness, long-term problems include periods of acute onset, often followed by periods of stability (plateaus) followed by further periods of activity.

The patient's attitude towards their illness

The experience of caring is closely related to the personality, character and attitude of the person being cared for (as well as their carer) and their attitude towards the disease. Consider the following attitudes or positions adopted by the carer and the person being cared for:

- stoical
- indifferent
- determined
- fatalistic
- angry
- accepting.

You may recognize your own attitude here. Do you also recognize why and where this attitude comes from and how it developed? Many media reports of illness experiences encourage the idea that we must fight disease. Have a look at these headings, used by newspapers to highlight illness experiences.

Young mum battles cancer
Brave teenager's fight against cancer
Fireman struggles with multiple sclerosis
Writer pits wits against cancer tumour
Never-say-die child fights against the odds

The 'take home' message from many of these statements indicates that people have a fight on their hands and that caring is about struggle. I can agree with that on one level – sometimes caring is a struggle, especially when you as the main care provider feel physically and mentally tired. Much depends on having a positive attitude and trying to remain as positive as you can, for both your own peace of mind and the person who often looks to you for inspiration.

The importance of a positive attitude

Is it any wonder that a common attitude adopted by people when they are diagnosed with a life-threatening illness is to see it as *a struggle against the odds*?

I use the term 'patients' (from *patiens*, 'suffer') to signify how people with illnesses are often referred to. Contemporary depictions of certain conditions, such as cancer, highlight a warlike picture with cancer *sufferers battling the disease.* Often we hear of the brave cancer *victim* depicted in warlike terms. These metaphors help to shape popular opinion about what it is like to experience certain diseases. Having an illness is like many other experiences; we learn to live with the many challenges that occur as a result of our situation. Our previous attitude towards problems, life events and crises helps to determine how we deal with major stress events. To a large extent, as the writer Susan Sontag (2001) pointed out, illness is a metaphor for behaving in a variety of different ways; much depends on what we are allowed to do. Metaphors that suggest we *suffer illness* accuse us of being passive recipients of many things that we can act against. Metaphors such as *victim* indicate a degree of servility, as if we play no part in our own health. In caring for someone with an illness, it is important to consider the impact that the image of illness has on the person experiencing the illness, as well as on the supporter. We have choices. Do we respond as a victim/sufferer, or as a person? The term 'person living with HIV/AIDS' (PWHA) denotes someone living with their altered lifestyle and is more neutral than a 'cancer victim' who has been victimized and is largely powerless. 'Cancer victim/sufferer' is a disempowering term. Do we have to suffer? Is it acceptable to be seen as a victim? A stroke *victim* suggests a person struck down suddenly, assaulted by this terrible disease. What we are not aware of is that the person may have experienced high blood pressure (a common predisposing factor) for many years, as well as other factors that would make them susceptible, such as being overweight, having a poor, high-fat diet and having experienced stress.

Positive thinking

For many, being positive about yourself is about feeling positive. One of the most common symptoms of being a carer is called *compassion fatigue*. This is closely associated with feeling mentally and physically tired. Moreover, it is a state of mind where you feel lacking in ideas, pessimistic about your abilities and experience low confidence and self-esteem. These episodes occur naturally for most people at different times, such as Monday morning, Sunday evening, first day back at work, when we feel daunted by the task(s) ahead of us or unable to work out what to do. These everyday thoughts and feelings can drain our energy and demotivate us to a point where we feel unable to do anything. One of the best ways of tackling this problem is to prevent these feelings occurring in the first place. Positive thinking can also help when we find ourselves fed up and lacking inspiration. The trick is to use your own thoughts and feelings about different aspects of life. For some, making a cup of tea helps (unless you run out of milk!). Talking to others is often very helpful and important; the Samaritans are a great organization and can be easily contacted in a crisis (see Resources, page 136). Here are a few quick and easy ways of jump-starting your thoughts and feelings.

- Follow the three Rs: respect for self, respect for others, responsibility for your actions.
- When you say, 'I'm sorry,' look the person in the eye.
- Smile when picking up the phone; the caller will hear it in your voice.
- Don't let a little dispute spoil a good relationship.
- Spend some time alone.
- Never interrupt when you are being flattered.
- Try reading more – it is better than TV.
- Teach yourself to speak slowly, but think quickly.
- Memorize your favourite poem.

Summary

This chapter has provided an outline of the carer's role. Being a carer involves sacrifice and giving up things in order to help someone else, and that someone else may be a spouse, brother/sister, mother/father, cousin or neighbour. I have outlined some of the personal attributes (such as compassion and empathy) that can enable the carer to fulfil the role and to feel a sense of satisfaction. As you reflect back on the chapter, you may have many thoughts: *Have I taken on more than I can handle? Will I, or can I, be a good carer?* The fact that you have made that initial first step to say 'I care and I will make a commitment' is a huge decision. Chapter 2 takes a closer look at some of the practical issues faced by carers each day in order to manage the day-to-day activities of caring for a person with a long-term illness. Some of them may not apply to you, but others will be very familiar. Remember to try and think positively and consider that caring is not an isolated activity, but one that others are doing every day. Above all, there is always help and support available.

2

Practical issues

Introduction

The purpose of this chapter is to focus on the practical issues that can occur when caring for someone with a long-term illness. I will try and cover most common problems using what many health care professionals call an Activities of Daily Living approach (ADL). This method encompasses a wide range of things, such as breathing difficulties, mobility and eating and drinking, which this chapter will focus on. To begin I want to reiterate that caring should not be an isolated activity. I will stress throughout the chapter the need for carers to define their boundaries at the outset and determine what you *can* do and what you need help with.

Sources of help

There are many available sources of support in the community that will help you. A particularly useful healthcare professional is the community occupational therapist (OT). The role of the OT is to assess a person's ability to carry out daily living activities in a range of settings. Primarily, in the home, many patients find it difficult to do things, such as get out of bed, wash and dress, use the toilet and make meals. As a carer, you will be involved in doing many of these things on the patient's behalf. Sometimes, however, you need to have help to do them and at other times you need to decide how beneficial it is to encourage the patient to remain independent. This is often where the role of the OT is invaluable, as they can advise you about the help and resources that are available and in what situations patients should be encouraged to carry out activities for themselves. Help is available from your Local Authority, known in some areas as the Social Care and Health Department or Social Services. In hospitals, ask for the Social Work Department. OTs play a key role in supporting people with long-term illness, especially people at home who need equipment to help them deal with day-to-day activities. OTs also support carers and have a vast range of knowledge about funding grants, useful resources and a wealth of understanding of the practical issues faced by carers and patients. Carers often face difficulties with patients who struggle with problems such as mobility, including getting up from a chair or bed, walking and transferring from bed to chair. These will be discussed in this chapter.

Mobility

For some people with certain long-term illnesses (such as MND or MS), being unable to get about unaided is a significant milestone in their illness. Not being able to get themselves around without help is often symbolic of the major loss of independence. This need not be the case, as there are so many aids to enable mobility, from Zimmer frames and glide-about chairs to battery-powered outdoor mini-cars (see Chapter 7 on getting help). Loss of mobility represents a challenge for the carer to consider how they can best assist the patient, but also to try to allow them to retain as much independence as possible. Chapter 7 also discusses the importance of retaining a sense of independence. Some people with spinal injuries may have started to accept their lack of mobility, while others whose mobility has slowly been eroded may still wish to struggle to do it on their own. Others with breathing difficulties, or with chronic arthritis, may have an inappropriate view of their ability to get about without help. In many cases, the person with a long-term illness may become tired and weakened by their condition and require appropriate assessment.

Key factors in maintaining mobility

Assessment

It is useful to consider having the patient's level of independent mobility assessed by a health professional such as a physiotherapist or OT. In certain cases a wheelchair assessment may be made and a referral to a wheelchair clinic advised. In other cases a range of aids, from walking sticks (after a stroke) to walking frames of many varieties, can be used depending on the type of problem, the person's ability, their future prognosis and the environment in which the aids are to be used. In certain houses wheelchairs may not fit through doorways and adaptations will need to be made.

ADL assessments

Comprehensive assessments of mobility can be included within what is called an Activities of Daily Living (ADL) assessment. These are often carried out before a patient is discharged from hospital following, for example, a stroke and include a home visit with the OT, physiotherapist and a nurse. At home these types of assessment can be requested by the patient, a relative, carer or district nurse/social worker. It is very useful to have this type of professional advice, as there are sometimes costs involved in obtaining aids for use in the home, such as bath seats. These assessments take into consideration more the patient's ability to get about, including getting in and out of bed, going to the toilet, bathing and doing things in the kitchen. Useful aids at home include raised toilet seats, bath seats and chair and bed raisers, to prevent falls and avoid excessive bending. A key issue relating to mobility and making changes to the home is the need to manage stairs and making appropriate adaptations to resolve this problem, which can be expensive. Aligned to this in some houses is the need for a downstairs toilet or for a chemical toilet or commode both of which can be discussed with the health professionals (OT, physiotherapist, district nurse) and obtained from Social Services or health and social care agencies.

What can friends and family do?

- Observe the patient for signs of fatigue, weakness and inability to do everyday activities indicating a need to assess mobility.
- Seek professional advice and assessment.
- Try to ensure as much independence as is practicable.
- Keep everyday things within the patient's grasp.
- Be vigilant about risk areas such as going up and down stairs and steps, for example, when going to the toilet.
- Make sure aids are used properly and well maintained.
- Prevent falls by anticipating risk from poorly placed mats and/or other floor coverings, as well as inappropriate heights of beds and chairs.
- If using the stairs or getting to the toilet is a problem, consider using a chemical toilet or commode and moving the bed downstairs, but get proper advice first and some help to move the bed!
- Be careful about using the bath and always use non-slip mats and devices to help get the patient in and out of the bath (ask the professionals for help about this).

Some of the things discussed in this section, such as moving a bed downstairs, will not be desirable to the patient and may be seen as an infringement of their personal space. As a carer, one of your key aims is to ensure the patient's safety at all times. Assessing the risks of falls at home including bathroom, stairs and toilet areas is an important consideration, as these are areas where many people experience difficulty. Being vigilant to these and asking for appropriate advice about prevention is a key way of showing you care. Helping the patient understand the need for change, and being sensitive to what the change means to them, will help to demonstrate your care.

Mobility problems become the focus of attention for many health care professionals. However, one of the key issues facing carers of patients with mobility difficulties is the associated problem of the patient becoming unable to walk due to breathlessness – a not uncommon complication associated with mobility.

Helping someone who has breathing difficulties

For a variety of reasons, being acutely short of breath is a very distressing situation for the patient and often for those with them. On a long-term basis the need for oxygen is basic to the maintenance of life. Preventing someone from becoming breathless is an important care factor. Anticipating their needs is key. For example, making sure things are placed within reach, such as comb, papers, food and drink, helps to avoid exertion. Providing assistance with getting on and off the toilet and moving reduces the need for oxygen and can help to prevent an acute respiratory crisis. It is important to understand that, with good knowledge and sensitive, informed reactions, many respiratory crises can be averted. The carer needs to keep calm and demonstrate common sense.

Fear

Carers of patients with breathing difficulties for any reason need to be sensitive to the fact that the potential of running out of breath is one of the most anxiety-provoking situations for anyone. Responding to the needs of breathless patients is extremely important, and lifesaving in some cases. Experiencing chronic respiratory problems such as Chronic Obstructive Pulmonary Disease (COPD), asthma or emphysema in itself can account for a lot of the anxiety associated with these illnesses. Carers need to know something about the way we breathe, and its control, in order to gain insight and sensitivity when dealing with breathless persons.

We breathe because the body has too much carbon dioxide (CO_2) (monitored by the brain), which it needs to excrete via the lungs. Our breathing therefore increases, we take in more oxygen and the excess CO_2 in the body is excreted via expiration from the lungs. The difficulty for people with long-term breathing difficulties is that they have abnormal, higher levels of CO_2 than others. They often have blue tinges around the ears and toes, and also normally feel cold at the extremities. We need to take care when giving breathless people with long-term respiratory problems too much oxygen, because of the danger of providing too much and effectively 'flushing out' their CO_2. This would mean their urge or 'drive' for breathing becomes difficult or is 'lost' and they will become distressed. Having said this, it is important that we do not *starve* them of oxygen. The key is to observe their breathing, especially their rate (how many times they breathe), rhythm (pattern) and the depth or quality of their breathing. As a general rule, improved breathing often involves an increased depth of breathing using the right amount of oxygen. Be aware that rapid shallow breathing indicates a need for more oxygen and a desire to get rid of CO_2. Watching the colour of the patient for signs of blueness (cyanosis) is a good indicator, and listening to what the patient tells you is also important! Many carers are able to determine when the patient is becoming distressed and will know that exertion of any kind, even just sitting them up in bed, can cause a breathless episode. Stress also causes breathlessness, which can be relieved by rest and reassurance – stay with them and hold their hand. The appropriate use of oxygen using the patient's mask or, in some cases, drugs such as Ventolin (Salbutamol), which helps breathing, inserted into a humidifier (a machine for delivering the drug via a small motor), will provide relief.

What can friends and family do?

- If the patient becomes suddenly breathless, ensure their airway is not obstructed.
- Encourage them to sit upright.
- If prescribed, give oxygen if their breathing becomes difficult – observe rate, rhythm and depth.

- Look at their colour and listen to what they say.
- Observe changes when giving oxygen – does the breathing improve?
- The comfort people receive from effective and sensitive care cannot be overstated. Holding a breathless person's hand can make a difference.
- Overcoming the fear of shortness of breath is helped tremendously if the carer remains calm and does not become distressed themselves.
- Anticipate difficulties and be aware of how exertion and stress can increase breathlessness.
- Never allow the patient's oxygen cylinder to become completely empty (order new cylinders in advance). Only administer drugs using machines if you are confident and experienced in their use.
- Educate yourself about the benefits and side effects of medication. In particular, monitor breathless levels using devices such as peak flow meters (which are tubes used to measure the amount of air expelled by the lungs) and, if you have one, a nebulizer. The longer-term use of oxygen is helped by moistening the oxygen received using a device known as a humidifier.
- Above all, call for help if the patient's breathlessness is getting out of hand and you feel the situation is becoming a crisis.

Eating and drinking

Central to maintaining good health is ensuring a proper diet. For most of us eating and drinking are closely linked with pleasure, so why would we not want this to be the same for people who have a long-term illness? The ability to eat and drink and enjoy doing so are important social and cultural indicators of health and well-being. Diet is an individual issue, and as a carer you may not always agree that the patient's diet is ideal, although certain principles determine the importance of having adequate food and drink to sustain health.

Ensuring adequate amounts of daily fluid can be very difficult, especially when going to the toilet is an additional problem and may unconsciously cause a reduction in fluids. This can be overcome by including foods rich in fluids in the diet. Appetite may fluctuate as the patient's condition progresses or because of lack of activity, the drugs they are taking or their state of mind. Like all of us, lack of appetite can result from feeling full, constipation or lack of desire. As a carer you will invariably have opportunities to prepare food with or for the patient and to assess their appetite, eating and drinking habits and weight.

Eating habits for people with long-term illness vary as much as content, although certain key issues can be said to be universal, such as the need for a balanced diet. Dieticians report that breakfast is the key meal of the day, with an opportunity to take important foods such as fruit, fibre, fluid and protein. Significant changes in weight should be observed; they can indicate excess eating or weight loss which can be symptomatic of an underlying pathology.

Key factors associated with healthy eating and drinking

To avoid them becoming the passive recipient of meals, try to involve the patient in planning meals, selecting food, shopping and cooking. If this sounds a bit idealistic, try to get them into the kitchen if possible, to smell and taste the food being cooked, as this improves appetite stimulation. Food and drink go together and, where possible, use alcohol wisely as an appetite stimulant before the meal. Remember the need to take medication with or just before food and be aware of any special instructions. Soup is a great standby and small amounts of good-tasting soup taken regularly may be the only way that food can be consumed. Don't forget to try something different once in a while.

Drinking adequate fluids (1.5 to 2.5 litres of water – more in hot weather; try ice cubes) is a major challenge especially when going to the toilet is an added problem. Small amounts of fluid (up to about half a cup) taken regularly will help to ensure adequate fluid intake, as well as provide interesting-tasting supplements such as herb teas, juices, fruits and ice cream. Avoid large volumes of fluid and excesses of beer and fizzy drinks rich in sugar. One of the first things to consider as a carer is to make a list, to find out what the patient likes and dislikes and what they have never tried. Avoid or include these wherever possible. By all means try to introduce new flavours such as ginger, but avoid garlic if this is a disliked food! Good food management (including preparing your own food) is essential to health. Appetite can be stimulated by preparation and diminished by slavish adherence to *food fascism*, where eating becomes a chore because it is full of restricted *dos and don'ts*. A key challenge to carers who are required to prepare food is to be innovative, mindful of restrictions but focused on what is likely to be eaten and enjoyed. There are many ways of encouraging a patient to eat and drink. For example, getting them to suck a few ice cubes to relieve a dry mouth or taking sample sips of juice (with added vitamin drops) all adds up to increased fluid intake and nutrients in the diet of a person who needs to improve their nutrition.

Helping the patient who cannot eat or drink

Eating and drinking are part of life's pleasures. For people who are unable to eat and drink unaided, as a carer it is important to ensure that we try to maintain this. I recall having to feed six patients at lunchtime on a ghastly psychiatric hospital ward many years ago. The focus then was on speed and consumption – the idea was to get as many of them fed as fast as possible and to return with an empty plate! I hope I have learned lessons from this. As a carer, it should be a privilege to help a patient to eat and drink. Consider the following steps as a way of preparing to feed another person.

- Let them know when the meal will be ready and what it consists of. This stimulates appetite physiologically and gets the juices going!
- Use napkins or another means of making sure that food is not left on the patient afterwards. Tissues are helpful, as are 'wet wipes'.
- Ensure food looks good and is not cold (unless that is what is required). Consider whether it is well proportioned and what the patient wants.
- Consistency is important if chewing food is a problem. Avoid pureed food unless it is necessary. Soup and ice cream are good standbys.
- Make sure you use appropriate cutlery – try not to use huge dessertspoons for a person with a tiny mouth.
- Offer food at the patient's pace – not too slow (it's frustrating if they like it), and not so fast that they cannot enjoy it.
- Engage in conversation. This is part of the social activity of enjoying meals.
- Ensure fluid is consumed (preferably water, as this is an ideal time to increase fluid intake). Avoid sugary drinks, which can bloat.
- Observe special precautions like patients with colostomies and when people do not have any dentures.

Loss of appetite

Loss of appetite is the most challenging problem a carer faces and can be related to feeling physically and psychologically unwell. The cause can be one of the following:

- feeling *overfaced by food* or put off by unappetizing tastes or smells
- constipation or indigestion
- sore mouth, oral infection or swallowing difficulties
- dislike of food, cannot taste or smell due to blocked-up nose cold /flu
- feeling sick/vomiting, food poisoning – caused by food or constipation

- effects of medication or treatment
- feeling depressed, anxious, tired and fed up.

Whatever the cause of the appetite loss, as a carer you need to find out what it is, how to alleviate it and how to prevent recurrence. It may be as simple as changing the mealtimes and portions to suit patients who only want a light evening meal and a bigger lunch. Making the food appetizing, serving it at the right time and in the right way are easier problems than food poisoning or medication effects. Swallowing problems can be remedied by making the food soft (seek advice from a dietician). Sore mouth problems can be overcome by using mouthwashes such as Corsodyl or cheaper sodium bicarbonate dissolved powder and glycerin/thymol mouth rinses. Fresh pineapple is also an excellent remedy for after-meal cleansing. Cooking smells can be offputting – try a bay leaf in green leafy vegetables to reduce odour. Dry food can be made moist by using mayonnaise or milk or other sauces. These can also be used to increase weight. Fizzy drinks can be added to tubes when feeding, to prevent obstruction.

What can friends and family do?

- As much as possible, try to involve the patient in the cooking, purchase and selection of foods (even if it means shopping online)!
- Ensure adequate fluid intake, and be aware of the patient's need to go to the toilet and what this entails. For patients who like alcohol, use it appropriately as an appetite stimulant and a means of getting pleasure from food.
- Make a list of favourite food and drink, making sure that this includes fruit, vegetables and drinks. Provide small appetizing food when the patient is hungry, and encourage fruit juice drinks as they stimulate appetite.
- Follow a recommended diet if one is prescribed – for example, patients with renal failure on restricted diets, diabetic or gluten-free diets.
- Keep meals interesting and try to stimulate appetite with

food supplements like bananas and other favourite foods.
- Plan mealtimes to coincide with times when the patient is really hungry.
- Avoid overfacing the patient with meals that are too large.
- Remember that being unable to feed yourself does not diminish the desire to enjoy interesting meals and drinks.
- When helping the patient to eat and drink, be aware of the timing. When offering food, consider dignity and respect and enjoy it as a social activity. 'Little and often' is a good maxim – regular sips of fluid or soup are sometimes better than a large meal.
- Keep an eye on the patient's weight – check weight regularly and report any fluctuations.
- If there is a need to increase weight, consider adding supplements to the diet.
- Consider asking for Meals on Wheels as a way of guaranteeing adequate meals for the patient.
- Remember to go out and enjoy social eating in public places. To avoid overfacing, children's portions can be requested. Discourage 'snacking' and keep foodstuffs (apart from fruit) out of the patient's sight.

Special feeding

Unfortunately not all people with long-term illnesses are able to enjoy food and drink the way most of us do, and require special assistance and the use of various devices to ensure adequate intake. These devices range from a relatively simple soft plastic feeding tube inserted through the nose and into the stomach (a nasogastric tube), or a thinner tube inserted just under the skin directly into the stomach (a PEG feed, or Percutaneous Entero Gastric feeding tube). In some very specific cases, a plastic tube like an intravenous fluid-giving line is inserted into a vein. This is called a parenteral feeding line (or total parenteral nutrition, TPN). These devices, which are sometimes used outside hospitals and operated by carers, provide nutrition to patients who for various reasons (such as being unable to swallow or not being fully conscious) require special measures of this kind. It is important that these tubes remain unobstructed, and special training should be provided to help you to appreciate and respond if difficulties arise. Despite these measures the principles outlined in this section – i.e. timing, preparation, dignity and respect and the social aspects of mealtimes – can still be adhered to. As a carer, it is important that you consider mealtime as a social activity. This will contribute towards the maintenance of a good daily routine as well as ensuring individual dignity and well-being. As I said earlier, eating and drinking is a pleasure that should not be restricted just because you have a long-term illness.

Supplements to the diet

For a variety of reasons some people need to increase their calorie and protein intake (lucky them!). There are a huge range of dietary supplements and food additives on the market. Calorie increases can be provided as puddings. Ask the patient what their favourite is and give them what they like when they feel most hungry. Here are a few of the commonly used substances that can be added to any diet according to the need to increase calories (if underweight) or to add protein.

- *Butter added to the meal in potatoes, pasta and vegetables.*
- *Whipped cream or creamer's soured cream and dried milk (to bulk the protein content).*
- *Mayonnaise and milk added to soups instead of water.*
- *Sugar added to cereal food and vegetables (such as carrots).*
- *Vitamin drops added to food. These are available from chemists. Check the dosage usually used for babies and use this if you are unsure.*

Your role as a carer, then, consists of being able to provide essential aspects of care such as helping the patient to eat as well as giving them assistance with other activities of daily living. This help may include intimate areas of daily living

– such as washing and dressing or going to the toilet – and requires skill, sensitivity and discretion.

Carrying out intimate aspects of care

As part of their role, carers are often required to carry out a range of intimate aspects of care – undressing the patient, assisting them in going to the toilet and helping with washing and dressing. This is part of the *art of caring* if carried out with skill and sensitivity. In this section, I wish to describe how carers can perform this important part of care with skill and sensitivity. At the same time, I discuss what this means in terms of establishing and developing a good relationship through the use of positive communication based on trust, mutual respect and personal dignity.

It is worthwhile considering the nature of the relationship between the patient and the carer and how this can affect the carer's role. As a carer myself, I was happy to carry out many aspects of intimate care when my father was ill and being cared for at home. Perhaps this was because I was a nurse and used to doing these things. However, it helped that my father was happy for me to do them because of our relationship. It is important, therefore, to consider the patient's feelings. You may, as the carer, be related to the patient. Does your father, mother, brother or sister want you to help them get dressed or carry out personal care, such as taking them to the toilet? It is useful to discuss these things in advance to see how both you and the patient feel about doing these things. In some, cases the patient may prefer a stranger, such as a nurse, to conduct aspects of intimate care. Some wives or husbands would rather a nurse or other professional carry out intimate aspects of care because they want to retain their relationship with the patient and not start doing things for them that would alter the way they have developed as a couple. It is always worth considering and discussing this if it applies to you.

Help with personal care: washing and dressing

How we feel is closely related to how we appear – in other words, our self-image (Lloyd-Williams 2004). Positive body image emanates from wearing personal clothes (or those that define our culture, such as wearing a sari). Our dress, make-up, smell, facial hair and outward appearance reveal things about how we are inside and are therefore very important if we are unable (because of illness, weakness and infirmity) to wash and attend to our personal hygiene.

Personal hygiene needs are of paramount importance and need to be considered every day. Do we shower every day or just strip-wash? Can patients decide not to have a wash? Yes, of course, ultimately the choice about personal hygiene is always one the patient makes, but it can be influenced by many factors, such as the amount of effort required to have a bath, shower or basic wash. Part of the skill of helping people with personal hygiene is to enable patients to make positive choices for themselves. Showering each morning can make one feel great, but not if it takes three hours, two people and a huge metal hoist and at the end you feel sweaty and exhausted. A basic wash using a sink or bowl can address the need to keep clean, avoid pungent body odours and look good. The extent to which carers become involved in washing depends on the patient's condition and their relationship with the carer. In some cases where the patient is physically unable to do certain things, such as reach their lower body or bend down, carers need to help them and in doing so make micro-assessments such as whether toenails need cutting (a job for chiropodists), whether they have a skin rash or a small wound (fistula) that needs attention. Helping patients wash intimate areas of the body requires tact ('Would you like me to help you wash down below?' 'Can I help you to wash under your breasts?'). Carers need to be aware of the intimate nature of such care and remain sensitive to the patient's needs, even if the patient appears to show a lack of inhibition, which may arise from time spent receiving institutional care from professionals. Discretion and tact play a very important part of retaining and maintaining a sense of dignity and self-respect. It is always useful to ask the patient how (and when) they want intimate care of this kind carried out. Providing choice, as a rule, is a good approach to use as a carer, as it enables the patient to feel that they have a part to play in their own care.

Care principles: washing and dressing

- The patient should be encouraged to do as much or as little as possible for themselves, according to circumstances.
- Adequate aids to assist with washing and using the bath/ shower should be in place, e.g. bath seats and grab rails.
- The end result is to maximize self-image and look (and smell) good.
- Men invariably may wish to have a shave (wet or dry).
- Women may benefit from occasionally removing unwanted facial hair.
- Good personal hygiene care can include washing, grooming of the hair, nails and skin, as well as ensuring cleanliness of genitalia.
- Patients with in-dwelling urinary catheters, stomas, wounds and wound drains and other invasive devices need careful and systematic care of skin around the area (take advice from experts and ask to be shown how to do this).
- Dressing patients with specific problems, such as limb paralysis following a stroke, can be a challenge. Carers should know or learn how to dress patients with problems such as spasticity (for example, putting the affected arm in a sleeve first).
- Choice of dress is important (clean personal clothes) and exercising that choice enables the patient to build self-confidence.
- Carers should encourage pride in appearance (using a mirror), especially for special occasions and the need for trips to the hairdresser's.
- Be vigilant in conducting intimate care, and report things you feel are abnormal (excessive dry skin, bruising, red or

broken skin, evidence of falling, painful joints). Inform a professional, family members, district nurse or the patient's GP.

What can friends and family do?

- If appropriate, have a washing and dressing assessment conducted by an occupational therapist. Seek advice on ways to adapt clothing (using Velcro on clothes or wearing loose-fitting clothes to aid dressing and to limit discomfort caused by excessive movement).
- Having dressing aids such as shoe horns and pick-up sticks can increase the patient's dressing independence and improve their physical ability.
- Make sure all bathing aids are safe and functional. Ensure that, as a carer, you are aware of the correct procedures for moving and that any equipment used in the bathroom to get the patient in and out of the bath work correctly and are well maintained.
- Make sure personal needs for hygiene are adhered to – for example, use of special soaps, washing at the sink, using a shower.
- Ensure clean personal clothing is always available and that soiled clothes are rinsed and washed.
- Identify preferred clothing – special types of material (for example, silk, linen) or any cultural dress codes – and adhere to them.
- Attention to nails is important (especially with people with diabetes) – seek a chiropodist's advice or ask a district nurse. Manicures, pedicures and hair-washing are very pleasant for *pampering days.*
- Ensure that bath aids and devices to assist with bathing and having a shower are properly maintained and fitted at all times.

Helping a patient go to the toilet

Going to the toilet is a natural everyday activity for us all. With the exception of those with colostomies (an opening from the internal bowel on to the abdomen) and those with a urinary catheter, the vast majority of people with long-term illness may need some form of help getting up for, or using, the toilet. The general principle that applies to all physical support is to encourage the patient to become as independent as possible and to provide help as required. In professional terms using the toilet stems from a knowledge that we need to open our bowels (or 'do a number two') at least once or twice a day, depending on our diet and level of mobility. We may need to pass urine at least five or six times a day, again depending on what we drink and environmental factors. We know that first thing in the morning, and after meals or drinks, are optimal times to go to the toilet and many people incorporate this into their daily routine. With some older people, their daily routine determines bowel habits, and not opening their bowels at certain times is indicative of a problem. As a general rule certain key factors can be established relating to bowel and bladder habits for people with long-term illness, especially those whose mobility are affected.

- Changes in diet and fluid intake, and changes to medication, can affect bowel habits and can also change the colour of urine.
- Dehydration, taking a lot of drugs, poor diet and a lack of mobility can cause constipation.
- Adequate fluid intake and a well-balanced diet help ensure regular bowel habits.
- Altered bowel habits and the presence of blood in the stool need investigating.
- Regular fluids throughout the day, especially water at mealtimes, should be encouraged (despite making the patient want to use the toilet).
- Walking to the toilet can be seen as a mild form of exercise.

- Changes in urine flow – especially amongst men – can be a normal part of ageing. However, being unable to pass urine, experiencing discomfort and passing smelly cloudy urine can all be a sign of infection or obstruction.
- Pain when passing urine, the presence of blood in urine and excessive trips to the toilet are abnormal signs and need investigating.
- Consider how some types of medication may cause a change to the colour of urine and/or alter bowel habits.

Looking after the carer

Helping a person to get to and use the toilet can involve a range of activities, from assisting them in getting up from a chair, to using a chemical toilet to using a stair lift. For the patient, getting to the toilet can involve the use of a range of walking aids, such as sticks, frames and wheelchairs, which are essential to ensure safety and to prevent falls. It is important that carers utilize all the aids available, including ceiling hoists, mechanical aids, chair raisers and grab rails. This will not only make it easier for the patient to move, but also prevent you (the carer) developing any problems such as back injury. It is also important to consider some of the safety issues involved in preventing accidents to carers and patients (discussed in Chapter 7), such as the removal of loose rugs and carpeting from toilet and bathroom areas. Research into the number and type of falls experienced by older people in their homes (Yardlley et al. 2006), suggests that loose rugs and failing to use mobility aids are key causes of injury to patients and their carers.

Summary

This chapter has covered some of the most difficult areas involved in being a carer. Central to a good quality of life is the ability to eat and drink. Not only is it a vital life activity but it is also an important social one. Ensuring that mealtimes (irrespective of the diet or circumstances) are sociable poses many challenges for the carer, especially if the patient happens to have breathing problems too! Planning meals, food preparation in the home, the expectancy of food and its consumption – all of these structure our daily lives. It is crucial to try and convey here that eating and drinking are important social rituals. Tablecloths, napkins, water (wine, perhaps) and conversation are all standard parts of the mealtime of many people (or should be). So why should people be left out just because they have a physical or mental long-term problem? In hospital, the long-term care of patients used to exist around mealtimes, with the ritual of toileting following the meal. The logic behind this is based on the gastro colic reflex, which stimulates bowel movement following the ingestion of food.

3

Managing pain and discomfort

Introduction

Caring for anyone with an illness or medical condition which makes them dependent on others creates a range of challenges for the individual patient and the carer. In this chapter I want to consider one of the most difficult challenges facing doctors, nurses and a range of professional and lay carers – pain and discomfort.

The chapter focuses on how to assess pain and discomfort, as well as looking at ways to relieve and hopefully manage physical discomfort. The issue of pain is vast and in some cases complex; the psychological aspects have been taken out and are considered in more detail in Chapter 5. I make no apologies for not offering any specific or immediate cures or long-term easy solutions. Rather, this chapter provides a set of guidelines based on personal and professional experience on how we might begin to assess, measure and determine what may be influencing the patient's experience of pain and discomfort. I also discuss some of the pharmacological and non-drug methods that can be used to control this pain.

The experience of pain

In modern times, major advances have been made in medical science generally, as well as progress in health care associated with controlling physical pain and discomfort. Despite this, physical pain and discomfort are major areas of concern for many people with long-term illness. The specific cause of the pain is not always known, although many can attribute their pain to activities they know affect it such as gardening or lifting. There is a well-known view in nursing circles which suggests that pain is a subjective experience and is *what the experiencing person says it is*. Despite this, anecdotal evidence suggests that many people have a hard time convincing health care professionals of the nature and intensity of their pain and discomfort. This may be due to the fact that different conditions result in different types of pain, or what is often referred to as *the total pain experience.* I think it is now useful to discuss origins and types of pain, causes and treatments. I will place emphasis on physical as well as psychological causes and treatment, as it is important to understand the link between the two.

People respond to pain in different ways, and pain experience can increase or decrease as a result of one or more of the following:

- The patient's culture (some people have higher levels of pain threshold, because they learned to express pain in different ways).
- Individuals' ability to tolerate pain (and what the pain means to the patient).
- Mood and morale.
- Physical pain is closely associated with the way we feel. When we are tired or anxious, we may experience more intense pain.
- Pain comes and goes and sometimes we become less tolerant to pain that never seems to go away.
- Drugs react differently in different people and responses to drugs vary because of a range of things such as body weight.

This list is incomplete and, as we all know, pain experiences alter daily (and in some cases hourly) according to our energy levels, sleep pattern and mood. Taking painkillers unfortunately does not always guarantee relief of pain and in some cases medication can make it worse! What is clear to doctors and nurses is the link between the way we feel psychologically and the experience of pain. It is important that we consider that, because pain is complex, we include how a person feels when working out how to help them. This is referred to as *total pain assessment*.

What can friends and family do?

- Listen carefully to what the patient is saying about the pain. What type of pain is it – sharp, dull or intermittent? On a scale of 1 to 10, how severe is it?
- Consider when it started. What were they doing? How long does it last?
- What effect, if any, has medication had?
- Does the pain become easier if the patient changes their position?
- What makes the pain worse?

Understanding *total pain*

Not all people with a long-term illness experience pain that may be defined as an *unpleasant sensory and emotional experience*. Indeed, 25 per cent of patients with cancer experience no physical pain (Twycross 2003). When assessing pain it is useful to consider that it involves not only the physical but also the social, psychological and spiritual dimensions of life and thus can be referred to accurately as *total pain* (Saunders 1970) (see figure 1 below).

What is pain?

Assessing pain

Because pain is individualized and complicated by so many other factors, it is hard to know what and when a person is experiencing pain. For example, many people with long-term pain may not look like they are in pain because of the absence

Figure 1: Assessing total pain experiences

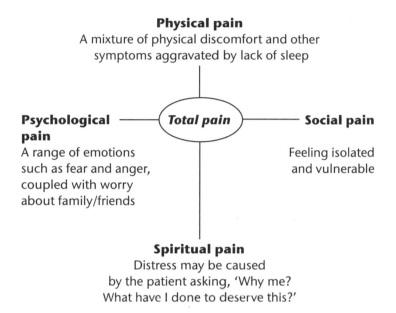

Physical pain
A mixture of physical discomfort and other
symptoms aggravated by lack of sleep

Psychological pain —— *Total pain* —— **Social pain**

A range of emotions
such as fear and anger,
coupled with worry
about family/friends

Feeling isolated
and vulnerable

Spiritual pain
Distress may be caused
by the patient asking, 'Why me?
What have I done to deserve this?'

of damage to tissues. Also, because they have managed to adapt to the feeling of pain, it appears to have become part of their physical everyday make-up. Equally, people with long-term conditions such as arthritis can experience different types of pain at the same time.

As carer of a patient who experiences pain regularly you need to know certain things about the patent and *their pain*. You need to know how to make an assessment of the pain in order to help make decisions about its severity, duration and whether medical help may be needed. One way of doing this is to use a pain scale. This is a simple 1 to 10 visual illustration, (see the *smily faces* in figure 2, p. 46). It does not have to be complicated or fancy. Above all, it must be understandable to you and the patient so that, even if the patient is unable to

Figure 2: Measuring pain experiences

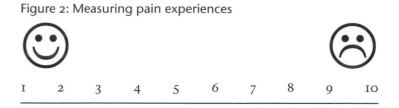

| I | 2 | 3 | 4 | 5 | 6 | 7 | 8 | 9 | 10 |

speak because of the discomfort, they can point out how their pain feels at the time.

It is useful to talk about different pain experiences when the patient is not experiencing pain. This way, you can try to understand how the pain affects them. Consider the different types of sharp sudden pain felt in the chest when experiencing angina (lack of oxygen to the heart) compared to the dull ache associated with sitting too long in one place. It is also useful to understand how one type of pain, such as indigestion, can differ wildly from, say, a headache or pain in the toes caused by cramp. Take a look at the list of types of pain below and on a scale of 1 to 10 indicate how much pain you felt. Compare this with another person, and discuss your different experiences of pain.

Type of pain

- toothache
- period pain
- labour pain
- migraine
- painful swollen joints (arthritis)
- renal colicky pain (stone trapped in kidneys, ureters)
- sprained ankle
- severe indigestion
- chest pain from angina
- trapped finger in a door
- broken leg/arm

How do we experience pain?

The experience of pain results from stimulation of various parts of our body – from our skin, muscles, bones, soft tissues and nerves via the spine, to our brain, where we make sense of the stimulus (which travels at different speeds) and come to associate the sensation as pain because it is an unpleasant feeling. Because the experience of pain is interpreted in the brain, it can also be experienced more intensely if the patient is worried or anxious about other things, for example, worries about family, money, employment or dying. Many people often worry that the pain is not going to be controlled, making the total pain experience much worse! On the positive side, relieving anxiety and fear by listening, staying with the person, holding their hand and providing reassurance through empathic statements such as 'It must be very difficult for you to experience pain every day', can relieve the patient's *total pain experience*.

What is experience of pain like?

Describing pain to another person is difficult, as it requires there to be almost a shared understanding of what the words mean., The following list gives us some idea of the things that go into understanding and treating pain:

- What is it like?
- What makes it better?
- Is it worse at any particular time?
- What makes it worse?
- How severe is it?
- What does it stop the patient doing?
- Is it there all the time or does it go away?

Preventing pain and management of pain require a broad approach. Some (physical) pain can be relieved by the use of drugs such as paracetamol. Other types of pain caused by compression of nerves may be a lot harder and require specialist drugs and medical intervention. Psychological and spiritual pain originating within the patient requires the carer to become aware of the concern and to give the patient permission to share their concerns and have them talked through in a sensitive way. Like physical pain, there may not always be a cure, but comfort and relief can be gained. In the process, a better understanding of what the patient is experiencing is likely to occur.

What can be done to prevent and reduce pain?

There are many ways to prevent and control pain:

- medication, including hormone therapy
- surgery (operations to nerves that convey pain sensation)
- radiotherapy (can be used to relieve pain)
- complementary therapies (a range of essential oils and massage)
- hypnotherapy, visualization and acupuncture (acupressure)
- TENS machines (giving a mild electrical stimulant to relieve pain sensation)
- providing information
- massage/heat pads
- relaxation and a range of psychological therapies
- specific pain interruption using local anaesthetic drugs (lignocaine and Entonox)
- modifying lifestyle, immobilization, avoidance of pain-inducing activities.

Progressive pain relief

The best approach to take with pain relief is to prevent it happening in the first place, by knowing what causes it and avoiding those activities where possible. Practically this may not be possible if the patient gets pain from doing everyday activities such as getting out of bed. In such instances, it is useful to anticipate the pain and provide appropriate antici-patory medication before carrying out the activity that causes the pain. Where possible, have a physiotherapist or occu-pational therapist give advice on ways to limit the exertion involved, or have aids fitted (such as bed or chair raisers or grab rails), to reduce the discomfort involved in moving (especially when dressing and washing). Relief from pain can be achieved by using all the available approaches.

Medication

There are some key principles involved in the use of drugs to prevent and control pain. These include using the three Rs: giving the *right* drug at the *right* time via the *right* route.

Most drugs in the UK are taken orally, including morphine and many analgesic (pain-controlling) drugs. That does not mean to say that other routes, such as patches, cannot be used. If the tablets cause gastric pain, consider alternatives and ask the patient's doctor for advice.

Different routes for taking medication

- oral (including sublingual, where the tablet dissolves under the tongue) or slow-release (SR) preparations, which give smaller doses over longer periods
- solution where the swallowing of tablets is a problem (Oramorph)
- lozenges (e.g. Fentanyl citrate)
- patches (such as Fentanyl), a morphine-based drug
- injection (useful for sickness where tablets are not toler-ated)
- suppositories, rectally (a quick method that includes morphine)
- via a nebulizer (morphine included, and Ventolin to relieve breathlessness)

Note: Avoid crushing medication and taking it out of the capsule, as this alters its action.

Using painkillers

The most common drugs used to relieve pain are a range of analgesics (painkillers), of which there are three categories:

- opioids (morphine-based)
- non opioids (paracetamol and non-steroidal anti-inflammatory drugs (NSAIDs)
- adjuvants (steroids, antidepressants, sedatives).

As a means of helping them determine the best type of drug to prescribe and administer, doctors and nurses in palliative care often make use of an analgesic ladder devised by the World Health Organization (WHO) (see diagram on p. 51). The basic idea is that drugs from each category are used appropriately in a broad way either as a single drug (such as paracetamol, which is a non-opioid drug) or used in conjunction with other drugs to maximize their effect. Most drugs have several effects. For example, paracetamol relieves pain but can also reduce temperature (i.e. it is anti-pyretic). Although a popular and well-used drug, it does not reduce inflammation, so is limited in the treatment of arthritis, which tends to be more responsive to anti-inflammatory drugs such as aspirin and NSAIDs. Unfortunately, many people are sensitive to aspirin which is excellent for reducing temperature, but has side effects causing breathlessness in some patients with asthma. Common NSAIDs include Diclofenac, Ibuprofen and Naproxen. These drugs work by reducing inflammation, although they also have many side effects, most notably gastric irritation, which is why some people prefer not to use them.

- Opioid drugs are morphine-based and include morphine, diamorphine (strong opioid), Fentanyl, Oramorph (morphine solution).
- Weak opioids include synthetic morphine drugs such as Omnopon.
- Non-opioids include paracetamol, aspirin and NSAIDs.
- Adjuvants include antidepressants, antibiotics and steroids.

Figure 3: The analgesic ladder (WHO 1996)

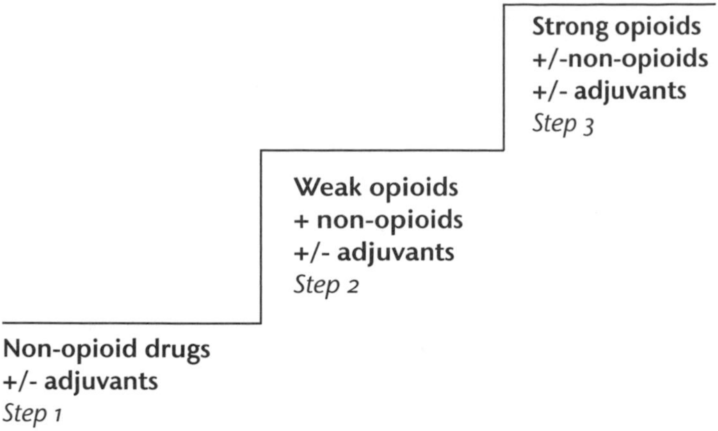

**Strong opioids
+/-non-opioids
+/- adjuvants**
Step 3

**Weak opioids
+ non-opioids
+/- adjuvants**
Step 2

**Non-opioid drugs
+/- adjuvants**
Step 1

How the ladder works

The ladder works on the basis that the patient is given the right individualized drug to relieve the pain and prevent recurrence. The dose is calculated in order to ensure optimal effect.

Step 1: non-opioids +/- adjuvants
At Step 1 pain relief could be achieved by paracetamol (two 500mg tablets) prescribed for joint pain every four hours. However, if this fails to work effectively within 24 hours, proceed to Step 2 by going up the ladder.

Step 2: weak opioids + non-opioids +/- adjuvants
Pain relief can be achieved by using a combination of parac-etamol and stronger non-opioids such as codeine or dihydro-codeine, with the aim of controlling the pain. The only reason not to give stronger drugs is if the patient does not tolerate them because of side effects. If the increased drugs do not cause the desired effect, then Step 3 is taken.

Step 3: strong opioids + non-opioids +/- adjuvants

At this step, opiates such as morphine (5–10mg), either slow release or tablets, can be used, or higher doses of Step 2 drugs such as two tablets of Co-Codamol, which contain 60mg of codeine. Consideration will be given to using morphine, as this can cause nausea, vomiting, constipation and adversely affects patients with kidney problems. If the patient's pain is controlled with the morphine and no side effects are experienced, the dose can be gradually increased every 24 hours until the pain is fully controlled.

Practical considerations about pain management

Managing pain is not easy, largely because of the uncertainty about what causes the pain as well as the many psychological factors that can influence the pain experience. Consider these practical tips to summarize what has been discussed about pain and its management:

- Try to find the cause of pain and treat or deal with this.
- Anticipate pain and provide anticipatory pain relief.
- Have drugs available for spontaneous or *breakthrough pain* (a flare-up of acute pain, moderate or severe, and usually of short duration).
- Provide regular analgesia as prescribed, but do not wake the patient up to take medication. Report side effects immediately.
- Use non-drug methods wherever possible, such as complementary therapies.
- Be aware of drug side effects and interactions between prescribed drugs and non-prescribed drugs.

Most painkillers such as paracetamol and morphine have side effects, the most significant of which is constipation. For this reason, when the drug is prescribed information about the side effects should be provided. Morphine, for example, causes nausea and should be prescribed with anti-sickness medication, or in some cases nurses will give an injection with each dose. Patients taking morphine or any long-term pain-killers should be aware that constipation can occur and a mild laxative or bowel regulator should be given. Better still, make sure the diet contains fibre and extra fluids to help the body metabolize and excrete the drugs.

Preventing pain

Good pain management includes knowing when to give what drugs. For example, if the patient experiences *persistent pain,* it is better to try to prevent the pain and give analgesics regularly and *as required. As required* medication is prescribed when it is clear that the patient's pain occurs outside regular times. A good example is a patient's recovery from surgery where the pain becomes intense after their usual doses of analgesia. In this case, *as required* medication is prescribed because it is required *above and beyond* regular painkillers. It is useful to have a back-up medication such as paracetamol (non-opioid), which can be given in between regular doses.

Non-steroidal anti-inflammatory drugs (NSAIDs)

These drugs are commonly used to control pain, as well as being used with opiates to achieve maximum effect. They are particularly useful against pain caused by inflammation, so are often used in arthritic conditions as well as to relieve pain caused by many cancer tumours. NSAIDs have been very effective over the years, although they have numerous side effects. Some of these side effects are experienced in a few drugs and only then in higher doses; others are common to most NSAIDs.

Common side effects of NSAIDs

● Fluid and salt retention and adverse effects on urinary system resulting in swelling around the ankles (oedema) and, in some extreme cases, renal failure. Be wary if taking diuretics (water tablets). Seek medical advice.

● Can cause gastric irritation.
● Nausea and vomiting.
● Can have an effect on the formation of some blood constituents (platelets).
● Aspirin can cause tinnitus and deafness.

Note: If in any doubt about the effects of any drugs seek medical advice.

Remember there are a lot of ways in which pain and discomfort can be relieved, including giving information and providing reassurance. Assessing and anticipating pain helps doctors and nurses to prescribe the correct medication. Total pain experience includes considering the way patients feel, how tired and anxious they are, as well as their level of self-confidence. As carers it is important to know how the patient is feeling as well as being aware of the action of drugs and what side effects they can induce. Above all, remain aware that pain is what the patient says it is and their total pain experience includes physical as well as psychological well-being. This process of moving up the ladder *does not continue* if the patient experiences unwanted side effects from the drugs.

Non-drug methods of relieving pain and discomfort

Drug therapy is often seen as the major way of treating pain in long-term illness, although many drug treatments work well in combination with non-drug methods of relieving pain. A number of non-drug therapies, as well as complementary therapies, have become popular and are used to treat pain and discomfort by providing relief and comfort. These include relaxation, aromatherapy, massage, reflexology, hypnosis, guided imagery, visualization and shiatsu, biofeedback and cognitive behavioural therapy (CBT). The latter is a psychological method of changing people's thoughts and enabling them to cope better with their situation (this is also discussed in Chapter 7, p. 118). In terms of pain relief, CBT can be used to help people to cope with their pain and discomfort to reduce suffering and enhance quality of life. Knowing about the illness can help the person and carer to know what can be done without resorting to the use of drugs. The most basic form of non-drug treatment is relaxation, which has been used as a therapeutic tool for centuries because of the relationship between muscle tension, stress and anxiety. It is well known that increased muscle tension can increase the experience of pain. Relaxation techniques can be learned and used. They involve learning to progressively relax skeletal muscle groups over a period of 20–40 minutes and are an integral part of other therapies such as yoga. Effective relaxation should take place in a quiet environment and has been known to cause comfort and aid wellbeing because it can distract the sufferer away from the pain (Horn & Munafo 1997).

Exercise

In some cases discomfort can be relieved by gentle aerobic exercise through the release of endorphins (natural painkillers). 'Aerobic' simply means 'with air'. When an exercise or activity is described as aerobic, it means the conditions allow your body to replenish the needed oxygen (air) to the muscles being exercised. Anaerobic exercise builds muscle and is needed to strengthen heart, lungs, immunity, lower blood pressure, maintain good cellular health and help prevent or control major diseases (like diabetes, cancer atherosclerosis, asthma, sciatica and emphysema). It can also help with the symptoms of some diseases, such as osteoporosis and arthritis, by helping to relieve discomfort. Depending on the type of pain and discomfort experienced by people with long-term illness, some can be relieved by gentle massage rather than using morphine-based drugs. Some discomfort is intermittent and is not always present. Other types of discomfort can be relieved by reliving a pleasant memory or event, or eating especially good food. Clearly if the pain is severe, it is necessary to use drugs for immediate relief, which is what pain medication is for.

What can friends and family do?

Taking medication to relieve pain and discomfort is important and in many cases vital to maintain well-being. Taking long-term medication can bring its own problems, such as dependence with morphine and inflammatory responses when using steroids. It is important to look out for signs of drug interaction, as well as to be aware of any new pain or discomfort that cannot be accounted for by the illness. All too often pain and discomfort can be seen as a sign of old age or as a part of the disease process. Friends and family need to be aware of any changes in the patient's condition that cause pain and discomfort and to report any of the following symptoms to a doctor or qualified nurse immediately:

● pain or discomfort, if it results from injury or a fall where the spine is injured
● pain experienced at night or at rest
● pain that radiates down arms and legs, or weakness/numbness in arms and legs
● pain that causes problems to bladder or bowel function
● a new pain that is accompanied by a rise in temperature.

Looking after the carer

This chapter has focused on the management of pain and discomfort. The experience of pain can often cause psychological as well as physical distress for the patient, but it can also have a detrimental effect on the carer. It is very difficult and worrying to be with someone who is in pain, especially if they are a loved one or a person that you are committed to caring for. It is important for you as a carer to feel that you are doing your best to help them relieve their suffering. It is also necessary that you receive adequate help, support and appropriate advice to help you gain the necessary self-confidence to care for the patient properly. To do this, try to have contact details of medical and nursing staff, as well as others who have agreed to help you and provide advice. Should you feel worried about your role in managing the patient's pain and discomfort, seek help from the GP, a nurse or a friend who is willing to support you, give a second opinion or share your concerns. Preferably, if the problem is a medical one, seek appropriate medical/nursing advice and if it is out of hours consider other forms of help such as the NHS help line.

Summary

This chapter has focused specifically on the relief of pain and discomfort. These important aspects of care need to be tackled as and when it occurs. In some cases, it is more effective to provide pain relief before pain occurs (such as when moving someone with a sore back worsened by movement); this can eliminate the experience of pain itself. While taking medication to relieve pain is important, this chapter has also considered non-drug treatments. It is sometimes necessary to consider that there is not always a pill for every ill, and that the cause and treatment of pain and discomfort can be found by simple activities such as relaxation, movement, exercise, massage or distraction. Over time, the pain and discomfort associated with long-term illness can wear you down physically and psychologically, leaving you feeling anxious and (in some cases) depressed. Physical pain is often easier to manage than its psychological aspects. Many people with long-term illness experience discomfort caused by feeling insecure, lacking in confidence and low in mood. We look more closely at this aspect in Chapter 4, where we also consider the activities that people with long-term illness can become involved in, as well as the role of the carer in helping the patient to maximize their activity and considering the best way of helping to improve life through activity. In Chapter 5 we consider the psychological needs of the patient and the important role carers play in providing support and guidance.

4

Specific activities of daily living

Introduction

This chapter focuses on those everyday things we do in life that we take for granted and are known professionally as Activities of Daily Living (ADL). In particular, it looks at a specific aspect of care described by many as the British disease – the so-called obsession with bowel and bladder problems. The fact that a whole chapter is dedicated to one particular aspect of physical function reveals the multitude of difficulties often associated with bowel and bladder function, such as diet, infection and symptoms associated with bowel disorders, like nausea, vomiting and constipation. The chapter will also consider a range of remedies, both pharmacological and non-drug methods. Bowel and bladder problems can (and do) cause severe physical problems, as well as some very significant psychological issues. Central to the effective management of bowel problems is making sure that a proper well-balanced diet is taken.

Diet

Physical difficulties can occur in anyone who has a medical condition, although they may be temporary and transient in some or recur regularly for others as an acute short-term problem. My nursing experience leads me to believe that bowel problems ranging from constipation to diarrhoea are a recurring problem for people throughout the world, young and old, irrespective of their health status. Older people in hospital and those who have long-term physical problems can also dwell on their physical difficulties, with a considerable amount of conversation taken up on the topic of bowels.

People with long-term illness who also have mobility restrictions are often prone to bowel problems due to lack of movement, which causes the bowel to become sluggish. This can be made worse by having to take medication for pain relief, for example. The vast number of drugs used to relieve pain and discomfort can also adversely affect bowel function because of their action in slowing down and controlling nervous sensation. It should come as no surprise to carers that comfort and well-being are closely related to having a regular bowel habit.

One of the key factors influencing bowel function is diet. Maintaining a balanced diet is an important way to stay healthy. A balanced diet is one that contains the correct intake levels of protein, carbohydrates (but not too many), fat, minerals, vitamins and fibre (five fruit and vegetables a day, so they say). Having well-balanced, regular amounts of protein, carbohydrate and fat also means having meals at regular times so that the body can ingest and digest food properly. We should perhaps remind ourselves of certain basic rules about diet.

- Eat regular meals at roughly the same time each day.
- Start the day with breakfast.
- Avoid going long periods without eating and overeating later in the day.
- Always consume water with your meal, as it helps food digestion.
- Avoid excessive snacks – sweet, sugary foods, fatty crisps and high-salt foods – especially if you are trying to lose weight.
- Avoid eating late in the evening and then going to bed (not allowing the body to digest and metabolize food).
- Try to make sure your diet includes plenty of fruit and fibre.

Those who have a special diet – such as gluten-free, diabetic controlled, dairy free or protein reduced – need to ensure they adhere to their diet and weigh themselves regularly (at the same time of day). Despite mobility problems, it is important to try and prevent bowel problems arising in the first place. Often the onset of illness caused by a lack of appetite and enforced rest can cause changes in bowel habit. Bowel problems in people with long-term illness can arise for many reasons, including:

- poor diet, (lack of fibre), obesity and lack of mobility
- lack of fluids (insufficient daily water intake)
- history of bowel problems and overuse of purgatives in early life
- specific difficulties such as short bowel problem, spastic colon or Irritable Bowel Syndrome (IBS)
- taking regular pain-relieving medication (such as paracetamol and morphine-based drugs
- following surgical operations of the bowel.

Assessing bowel problems

Assessing bowel problems requires skill and some detective work! Often doctors and nurses will ask:

- What is your usual bowel habit?
- When did this pattern change?
- What medication have you been taking?
- When did you last have a normal bowel movement?
- Have you noticed anything different about your stools, such as changes in consistency or the presence of blood?
- Have you had any recent bouts of diarrhoea or urinary incontinence?

In some cases bowel habits change because of a change in diet, as a result of being hospitalized or changes in what you eat. In other cases bowel habit alters because of physical or psychological changes such as depression, causing a lack of appetite. It is not uncommon for some people to refuse to use toilets because they are unclean. In hospital some patients do not find it easy to use the toilet because of lack of privacy, or because they are too far from their bed.

Constipation

Some people have bowel problems that they have lived with for many years, as a result of poor diet or overuse of purgatives. Others suffer from constipation on a long-term basis and often regularly take suppositories or enemas. People with chronic-type constipation require regular attention from the nurse or GP. In some cases, the nurse may teach the carer how to carry out the procedure of giving the patient a suppository or enema, or in some cases the patients may be able to do it for themselves. However, if they feel embarrassed or have physical difficulties in doing it for themselves, a nurse or carer could do it for them. Bear in mind that, when it comes to intimate aspects of care, it is *always* worth checking out with the patient what they would prefer.

Giving a suppository

As with all aspects of care, it is important to explain what you are going to do. Preparation is important in terms of preparing the bed space, lying the patient on their right side with a waterproof disposable cover underneath in case of accidents. Ideally, they should be as close to the toilet as possible or have a commode nearby. Suppositories are inserted into the rectum using slight pressure and with some lubrication such as KY jelly. The suppository is inserted high into the colon (this may be difficult if there is bowel obstruction). Do not force anything into the rectum, and if the patient is experiencing severe difficulties ask for help from the nurse or doctor. Suppositories dissolve in the bowel and their action is to cause bowel movement within 10–15 minutes after insertion. Staying with the patient is helpful and necessary if they have mobility problems in getting to the toilet. Once they feel the urge, they should try and hold on for as long as possible, but not at the expense of having an accident on the way to the toilet. Afterwards, check if the suppository worked. Did it come back out? Ensure good hygiene by hand-washing and cleaning the patient, if necessary. In some cases, suppositories are a necessary way of getting the bowel working properly again. In severe cases it may be necessary for a nurse or carer to insert an enema. This medication works higher up the bowel and is administered using the same principle. Neither of these medicaments are a substitute for a proper, well-balanced diet containing plenty of fruit, fibre and water. Suppositories and enemas should not be seen as normal treatments for bowel problems.

What can friends and family do?

- Ensure the patient has a well-balanced diet.
- Try to eat meals regularly at roughly the same time each day.
- Make sure the diet contains fibre, fruit and vegetables and encourage fruit to be taken as snacks, rather than chocolate or high-fat and high-salt snacks.
- Drinking cups of hot water/ tea and including porridge for breakfast are good ways of stimulating bowel activity (as are small amounts of alcohol prior to meals – check which drugs the patient is already taking and possible interactions).
- Proper use of medical supplements, e.g. Fybogel as prescribed, to aid bowel movement.
- Encourage mobility (or passive leg exercises, if immobile) wherever possible, even if it is only walking across the room or standing up every hour.
- Encourage going to the toilet after meals to encourage regular bowel habits.
- Avoid too many stodgy foods and those rich in fats, such as red meat.
- Ensure the patient has an adequate daily fluid intake. Taking sufficient amounts of fluid (approximately 1.5 litres per day – ideally water) helps to ensure effective bowel function.
- If in doubt, seek advice about bowel problems and be observant for changes in bowel habits, such as frequency or changes in stool consistency.

Severe problems

In some cases where the patient has a long-term bowel problem – perhaps as a result of spinal injury, making the person immobile – severe symptoms can occur, including nausea, vomiting, stomach pain and discomfort. Chronic constipation can also make you very irritable and out of sorts, and occurs because the bowel has become obstructed or impacted. This can lead to the person being unable to digest food properly and hence feeling nauseous, and in some extreme cases vomiting (which can contain faecal matter). Investigations of these problems using X-rays reveals bowel obstruction. Such cases arise when the patient has not been mobile for many months or years and their diet has been poor. In extreme cases, nurses carry out what is called digital examination and manual evacuation of the bowel using the fingers. This is an unpleasant and uncomfortable procedure for anyone to experience and is often used as a last resort in conjunction with enemas and suppositories, often when these have initially failed to work. Digital evacuation should be left to qualified nurses to carry out. It requires a nurse physically removing impacted faecal material in order to relieve the symptoms and enable the patient to take a normal diet. In some cases, it is necessary to carry out this procedure on a more regular basis. To prevent this occurrence, the use of laxatives and bowel regulators is recommended (see box below).

Natural remedies to prevent constipation

The box below illustrates some natural ways you can prevent constipation just by including substances such as fibre to the diet. Patients who need to take regular painkillers and other drugs that slow down gut motility may invariably develop a sluggish bowel and over time may develop as a result of constipation. In itself, there is no real need for specific medication, although in some cases bowel regulators may be prescribed (many such products can be bought over the counter).

Medication may control constipation in a variety of ways. Purgatives, for example, tend to help increase bowel movements, whereas other drugs help to soften the stool and make defecation easier. It is advisable to seek professional advice in order to receive the most effective form of treatment, and bear in mind that many drugs can interact with drugs the patient is already taking. In some cases, where constipation is a minor problem, increased mobility such as a gentle walk, extra fibre and fluids should compensate if the patient has to take medication that slows down bowel function.

Natural remedies to prevent constipation

- Fruit* such as prunes (with/without custard). Syrup of figs, rhubarb and dates also act as natural aperients.
- Hot drinks (water, tea, coffee) tend to stimulate bowel movement first thing in the morning and after meals.
- Hot porridge at breakfast.
- Fruits, dried or fresh grapefruit, fruit juices and grated carrot added to soups.*
- There are also a number of natural remedies, such as cascara, butternut and blackthorn, that act as gentle laxatives and are found in many different brands.

* Patients with colostomies/ileostomies should avoid certain fruits and foods. Also, those with a history of bowel obstruction or bowel cancer should avoid eating fruits and pith.

Diarrhoea

Another common bowel problem faced by many people with long-term illness, and closely linked with constipation, is diarrhoea. This can result from having an impacted bowel and be a symptom of chronic constipation. As such it is not 'proper' diarrhoea, but is known as constipation with overflow. This is because the faecal matter obstructs the bowel, allowing only fluid to pass out of the rectum when the patient goes to the toilet. Other more common causes of diarrhoea include:

- infection (commonly salmonella) and poor hygiene caused by not washing hands before and after handling food.
- other conditions such as spastic colon, Irritable Bowel Syndrome (IBS).
- ingesting substances likely to cause gastric irritation, including foreign objects, alcohol or some prescribed or non-prescribed medications.
- eating foods not common to the diet, such as spicy curries.

If the diarrhoea persists after 48 hours, it is advisable to seek medical or nursing help. In particular, be sure to look out for signs of dehydration, especially if the patient is a small child or frail and elderly. In some cases, it may be useful to obtain a specimen in an airtight screw lid container (available from the GP), as this will help to determine the cause. Here are some important signs to look out for if dehydration is suspected.

- complaints of being thirsty
- dry mouth and mucous membrane
- dry, inelastic skin (in chronic situations, also sunken eyes)
- lethargy, listlessness (mild confusion in older people)
- passing little urine or dark, concentrated urine

What can friends and family do?

One of the most important practical things family and friends can do with any bowel or bladder problem is to ensure there is adequate access to the toilet and that the patient feels secure using it (and that involves having privacy). Lacking confidence in going to the toilet is one of the reasons why some patients in hospital become constipated because, for example, there is an inadequate lock on the door. If a patient does have diarrhoea or is constipated, it it vital that they drink plenty of fluids. This will help to replace lost fluids as well as easing their discomfort. In all cases, it is wise to try and estimate the amount of fluid lost due to diarrhoea. You may have to judge this by noting when they last went to the toilet properly. Make sure that the patient's anal region does not become sore and dry by keeping the area clean, and applying creams such as lanolin to prevent skin breakdown.

What can be done for the carer?

I keep mentioning prevention, but when caring for a person with diarrhoea it is important that the carer ensures a high standard of personal hygiene, particularly a good hand-washing technique. This helps to prevent the spread of any infection (if this is the cause). The carer may be washing the patient's anal region, applying creams to prevent soreness, and therefore needs to make sure they wash their hands thoroughly each time. Carers are advised to wear a plastic apron when carrying out tasks involving the bowels and bladder to prevent the spread of any infection on to their clothing. When finished, dispose of all equipment in a black bag and make sure it is incinerated. If you develop any symptoms similar to the patient, take a specimen to the doctor, increase your fluid intake and ask to see your GP if symptoms persist for more than 48 hours.

Good hand-washing technique

It is worth noting here the importance of good hand-washing habits. These can help to reduce cross-infection by as much as 10 per cent.

- Wash hands when you know you will be touching the patient's skin and are likely to pass on any bacteria from your hands to their body.
- Apply soap to hands, wrists, between fingers and over both palms and wrists.
- Rub soap thoroughly into the skin for one minute.
- Place hands under hot *running* water, rubbing in between and up and down the fingers.
- Make sure nail beds are clean and nails kept short.
- Rinse off all soap and repeat soaping and rinsing.

- Make sure the hands are dried – using either disposable paper towels or a clean hand towel.
- Make sure hands are thoroughly dry, and use cream to prevent dryness and soreness.

Colostomies and ileostomies

Long-term illness can include living with a colostomy or an ileostomy (both known as a stoma). These are artificial openings from the small bowel (ileostomy) and large bowel (colostomy), which allow faecal matter to pass into a plastic bag attached to the skin by strong plaster material. Stomas are surgically formed due to problems such as tumours or other obstructions in the bowel. Although a cause of stigma initially, after a while people with stomas often manage to cope with them quite well after the operation, learning about diet and changing and using different types of bags. Both types of stoma bags are supplied according to the maker's systems and the patient's needs. Ileostomy bags tend to fill up quite quickly and can be emptied using a clip rather than having to remove the whole bag. People with stomas can experience some skin problems around the area of the stoma, as the skin reacts to the substance used in the adhesive material that sticks the bag to the skin. Specialist nurses (stoma nurses) provide advice and information in hospital and at home about the different types of bag systems to use. People with stomas are advised to be careful about eating certain types of food that are likely to cause problems, such as onions (these are often mentioned). Carers may become involved in helping a patient to change the bag in certain circumstances, such as when the patient is unwell, although it is the patient themselves who should be encouraged to become independent in this!

The principles involved in stoma care are as follows:

- Carers/patients must wash their hands before and after changing a bag.

- Have a new bag ready for changing in advance.
- Ensure the bag fits well.
- Dispose of the old bag and note contents for signs of change in bowel habit.

Nausea and vomiting

Feeling sick and vomiting are dreadful symptoms that cause distress. They can also lead to weight loss and dehydration, making patients feel tired and anxious. Causes of vomiting vary from eating infected food to high levels of calcium in the blood (hypercalcaemia). It is also as a side effect of cancer treatments. In some cases, vomiting results from injury to the brain. Whatever the reason, it is important to find the cause and treat it, but also to relieve the distress.

Possible causes of nausea

- anxiety and stress
- constipation
- indigestion, reflux from a sliding hiatus hernia
- taking medication such as painkillers and non steroidal anti-inflammatory drugs (NSAIDs)
- anti-cancer drugs and antibiotics
- a build-up of chemicals in the body resulting in damage to the liver and kidneys

Many episodes of nausea and vomiting subside after 48 hours and may not require medical help. In some cases, specimens need to be obtained. It is useful to try and estimate the amount of fluid lost by vomiting, as it is a way of working out how much needs to be replaced. Estimating loss can help in deciding if the patient needs an intravenous infusion of fluid or whether they can best have it replaced by drinking extra fluids or having medicaments such as Reydrat. It is also useful to get an indication of what the vomited material is like. For example, dark brown suggests that it may have come from bleeding in the stomach, while a bright-red colour is more suggestive of blood from the lungs. Making a clear observation can help doctors decide on the best course of action. Feeling sick is unpleasant and patients often require psychological support as well as comfort care in the form of mouthwashes (to freshen the mouth and prevent the development of sores).

What can friends and family do?

When someone feels sick, there are some good, practical things that can be done. It is helpful to have a bucket or some receptacle ready in case they are sick. This should be clean and emptied if they are sick and replaced before you take the old one away – as a patient it is reassuring to know that there is always something to be sick into! Provide comfort by ensuring mouthwashes are available and given after being sick. Mouthwashes such as Corsodyl help to keep the mouth clean. Offer fluids as much as possible without making the patient feel worse. Little and often is a good maxim. It is important to keep the level of fluids up, even if it means sucking an ice cube. Once they are able to tolerate food, soup and bread are useful, if this can be tolerated. Avoid greasy foods and give the patient their favourite foods or anything they especially like. In older people and small children, who become dehydrated very quickly, severe vomiting can lead to dehydration very quickly, especially in hot weather.

In severe cases, medical help and hospitalization may become necessary. Some cancer patients experience nausea before their treatment, as well as after their chemotherapy (anxiety-induced). Specific things to do include:

- Offering anti-sickness medication as prescribed, before the sickness kicks in. Avoid giving tablets if this makes the patient sick. Medication can be given dissolved in fluid, suppositories or by injection.
- Try to identify if there is any pattern to the sickness. Does it happen before certain foods, at certain times or after medication?

- Avoid foods likely to cause sickness, but encourage dry foods, and *never* stop offering fluids to replace what has been lost.
- Avoid contact with food smells caused by cooking, as this can be very distressing.
- Long-term sickness often caused by cancer-related disease can be helped by complementary therapies such as relaxation, distraction, hypnosis, acupressure and acupuncture).

Carers should be aware that some herbal alternatives and remedies for nausea can interact with conventional medication. Consult your GP if in doubt about using nonproprietary medication for people with long-term problems and any possible side effects from using different drugs.

Skin problems

Skin problems arise in people with long-term illness for many reasons. Having clean healthy skin is important (especially in the face), as it influences self-image, well-being and self-confidence. Having healthy skin and being given good skin care can help to prevent as well as relieve symptoms and stop the distress of having red, sore and itchy skin. Part of this care involves a good level of personal hygiene. It is when washing and grooming the patient that many skin problems are detected. Skin breakdown often occurs as a result of a lack of movement. It can also occur because the patient has been moved, which causes pressure and friction. The skin will suffer if there is a lack of moisture and dryness occurs, or when there is excess pressure placed on bony prominences such as the elbows, hips, heels and the sacral area at the base of the spine. Problems arise when the patient is unable to move for long periods, and pressure and heat builds up. It is also made worse by a loss of weight or if the patient is overweight and dehydrated. Such problems are compounded by a range of factors such as illness (anaemia), starchy bed sheets, excess sweating, and urinary and faecal incontinence. All of these can give rise to the development of what is known as a pressure sore or decubitus ulcer. This is the breakdown of the skin in certain parts of the body due to excess pressure. Pressure sores are also caused when:

- there is a low level of circulating oxygen in the blood, such as when the patient has anaemia.
- lack of fluid and a poor diet lacking in iron.
- excessive pressure placed on hips and sacrum due to prolonged bed rest (such as when a spinal injury occurs).
- excessive weight loss or excessive weight.
- the patient has neurological problems, spinal injuries, dementia, and people who are on bed rest with reduced mobility.
- the patient is immobile and urine incontinent.

Many pressure problems are relieved by careful moving and handling and by sensitive consideration given to the micro-climate – the area affected by pressure. This can involve using non-starched sheets, ensuring adequate fluids, and making sure the patient is kept dry and clean at all times. Family and friends can make a huge contribution to preventing pressure sore development by paying attention to movement and ensuring that the patient's position changes regularly. Check if the patient needs the toilet and encourage a diet rich in vitamins and mineral supplements such as folic acid (prescribed by the GP in some older people). As mentioned earlier, it is also important to ensure the patient is not constipated, as this will add to the discomfort, as well as increase pressure in the sacral area.

Jaundice

Jaundice is a symptom and not, as many people describe, a disease. It results in yellowing of the skin and whites of the eyes, and itchiness of the skin. It is often caused by a problem with the liver, pancreas or gall bladder (which stores bile), and is frequently a symptom of certain types of cancer (cancer of the liver, for example). Jaundice can also occur as a side effect of some medications and as a result of blood transfusions, causing hepatitis (inflammation of the liver). Being jaundiced makes you feel very tired and unwell and in many cases the patient and carers may not realize that the patient's skin is changing colour slightly. Skin changes occur slowly over time and are hard to detect at first. The best way to manage jaundice is to find the cause and treat it with a healthy diet and appropriate medication for the cause. Skin colour will return to normal, although it will take a long time and can be very worrying to the observer and patient (avoid mirrors – it helps!).

How do you know if you have jaundice?

The following are known risk factors:

- previous history of hepatitis, liver disease not necessarily related to alcohol
- recent foreign travel
- medication given outside of the UK to treat an infectious disease
- vaccinations and treatment for hepatitis
- history of intravenous drug use or sharing needles
- recent blood transfusion
- feeling tired, lethargic and having itchy skin.

What can friends and family do?

People with jaundice often look very ill, although they seem reasonably happy in themselves. They tire easily and need a good diet, eating little and often. Family and friends should ensure that the patient takes their prescribed medication and avoids alcohol, and they should provide relief for symptoms, such as itching, especially around the anal region. Creams can be prescribed and bought over the counter for this. Sometimes abdominal swelling (Ascites) can occur related to liver problems. The extent of swelling needs to be measured regularly, as it causes alarm for the patient, who can look pregnant. The patient can feel very fed up due to itchiness, lack of sleep and feeling lethargic. Regular blood tests are often taken, which can be painful if the patient is unwell. Above all, it is necessary for friends and family to provide psychological support. Many symptoms occur and changes in the body can give rise to anxiety. These include changes to the patient's stools, which turn pale, float in the toilet and are very smelly. This is due to a lack of bile. Moreover, the patient feels very tired all the time, which is a major problem. This is often compounded by a lack of sleep and being awake at night because they have dozed off during the day and lie awake worrying about what is happening to them.

Resting and sleeping for patient and carer

An essential part of good health is ensuring that you get a good night's sleep. Night-time care for a person with a long-term illness can be a major source of concern often because carers need their sleep and cannot provide continuous 24-hour care. If the patient requires help at night because of breathing problems, going to the toilet or changing their position to relieve pressure, it is worth considering getting additional help at night from a night sitter (ask the district nurse or GP). Night sitters are often paid unqualified or qualified nurses who stay up and attend to the patients needs during the night. They are expensive to employ and may stretch the budget. In some cases it may be worth considering providing support on a part time basis. Night sitters – for example, from Marie Curie Cancer Care – are available free for a short period from the cancer charity if the patient has cancer. A good night's sleep is vital for both patient and carer.

What can friends and family do?

Achieving a good night's sleep is encouraged by:

- avoiding sleep during the day
- having a comfortable bed and mattress
- not being disturbed at night or being unduly worried
- avoiding alcohol just before bedtime (although this seems to be a way some people get to sleep)
- avoiding eating and drinking fluids just before bed
- having appropriate prescribed medication to help induce sleep
- having incontinence pads in place should problems occur in the night
- having urinary aids easily available and accessible by the bed
- avoiding certain medication before going to bed such as diuretics.

Remember that a good night's sleep is also required by the carer. Disturbances outside the house should be avoided. Sleep-related problems should be given priority as sleep is a habit, and once poor habits are adopted it is often very difficult to change them, such as early-morning waking at 3 a.m. or 4 a.m. To induce sleep, try having a hot drink in the evening; placing drops of essential oil (ylang ylang) on the pillow; or relaxation and deep breathing just before going to sleep. Reading can help some, but other people can carry on reading for hours! Sleep is more likely to occur if you have less to worry about!

Summary

Carers need to remain vigilant and focused, not just on managing problems as they arise but also preventing them taking place. For these reasons, issues such as eating and drinking should always be regarded as important, simply because they can lead to other problems fairly quickly, like dehydration, constipation and discomfort. Above all, when caring for someone who has difficulty eating and drinking or going to the toilet, it is essential to remember that the patient's dignity and self-respect can be compromised if carers forget that these things are personal. It is all too easy to forget the person when you are focused on a task that you carry out many times a day. Carers are able to develop the skill of making difficult tasks appear easy, simply because they can combine psychological support and care when carrying out important physical functions with the patient. In Chapter 5 we consider the psychological needs of the patient and the important role carers play in providing support and guidance.

5

Providing psychological support

This chapter will focus on the need for carers to provide effective psychological support. There is a growing body of research and knowledge that highlights the importance of carers in all areas of health care – be they nurses, doctors or lay carers – to use good communication skills in providing quality care. The chapter will focus on how these interpersonal skills can be used to enable the patient to express their concerns and receive empathic responses from the carer that will help to meet the patient's psychological needs, relieve distress and provide them with the necessary self-confidence to feel able to make decisions for themselves. Throughout the chapter I will use case-study evidence to show how important it is for carers to be able to listen to the patient, identify their emotional needs and make appropriate responses. In particular I consider the growing problem of patients with a range of neurological problems, specifically confusion, and I highlight the need for understanding, tolerance and empathy in relation to people with this type of problem. Moreover, the chapter examines situations where carers need to consider that the patient may be showing early signs of dementia, and discusses how to identify key signs and seek specialist intervention. The chapter also assesses the needs of the carer and discusses how to avoid becoming too stressed by your role, as well as compassion fatigue and burnout.

Psychological care

Caring for person involves a commitment to providing good physical as well as psychological care. The latter is a growing concern in the UK, as the Department of Health has pointed out that NHS patients, particularly those with cancer, are complaining about the poor levels of communication and absence of psychological care in many hospitals and hospices (DoH 2000). Not meeting a person's psychological needs can lead to anxiety and become a regular problem, leading to depression and affecting physical and psychological well-being. A number of authors have also pointed out that psychological care is linked with poor communication and the inability of health care workers to communicate effectively with patients. Psychological care is about maintaining the well-being of the patient and family (Skilbeck & Payne 2003; Becker & Gamlin 2006). People with long-term illness often undergo a wide range of emotions that cause distress that are unrelated to the physical condition. As a consequence carers may be unaware of the anxiety being experienced and the unexpressed concerns, unless they know the person well and invite them to discuss their fears. Consider the following scenario.

Case study: Jean

Jean (27) is a carer for her mother Cathy (58), who has advanced multiple sclerosis (MS). Cathy is referred to a consultant at a neurological clinic specializing in urology for assessment of her urinary incontinence. She has seen many specialists over the years but seems particularly tense and uncomfortable about her latest appointment. Jean notices her mother's anxiety and asks about her discomfort. Her mother bursts into tears in the clinic and explains that the specialist is the same one who treated her sister, who died when she was 26. Cathy recalls going with her for the appointment – the doctor was insensitive and made her sister cry. Knowing this, Jean has a word with the consultant prior to the interview. The consultant is grateful and acts in a very sensitive way towards Cathy, explaining about her urinary problems and discussing what options are available to her.

Eliciting concerns

In Cathy's case, her daughter could see the concern and responded with sensitivity. In other cases, people often hide their feelings or mask their concerns due to feelings of guilt, embarrassment or lack of confidence. It is always useful to be self-aware as a carer, as you may not realize the numerous concerns and worries of people with a long-term illness. Research informs us that many cancer patients have unexpressed worries about cancer recurrence, spreading the disease to their children or numerous feelings of loss associated with the disease (Fallowfield & Jenkins 1999). Others, with MS, dementia or MND, experience similar feelings of loss due to incontinence, loss of independence or low self-esteem (Buijssen 2005). Acknowledging that such concerns, worries and anxieties may arise due to a relatively trivial (to the carer) issue is a good start. It is also worth considering that, if ignored, such concerns can develop into a range of problems, such as panic attacks, phobias of going outside (agoraphobia), mood fluctuations and depression. There are many ways to help someone with anxiety, including getting to know them and becoming familiar with their concerns and worries. Showing concern for their welfare and expressing a genuine interest in their well-being by asking them how they are feeling. Taking note of their feelings, asking, 'How are you feeling in yourself?', getting them to articulate their concerns and worries and, importantly, *actively listening* to their concerns are all key skills.

What can friends and family do?

There are many useful practical and emotional things friends and family can do to support a patient experiencing psychological problems. Most of these stem from actively listening and trying to spend quality time with the person, without having a specific task to complete. In particular:

● Make good use of eye contact and express genuine understanding.
● Avoid making value judgments.
● Reflect on what the person has said, acknowledge their concerns and ask how they feel about the situation being described.
● Clarify the issues expressed and summarize or paraphrase the content.
● Make appropriate empathic statements: 'That sounds like it was difficult for you'.

Active listening is not as easy as it sounds and requires skill, patience and a genuine concern for others. It is important to consider that you are not responsible for their feelings, which can be changed often (if it is appropriate) by the people doing something for themselves. This can include taking actions to alleviate their worries (other than talking about them, which is a very positive step), asking others for help (such as a counsellor) or contacting other agencies – for example, GP, district nurse, housing department, social services – for advice. Consider the importance of people doing things for themselves, such as seeking and being provided with proper information. This can be both therapeutic and practically rewarding, as well as good for improving self-confidence. Carers should *avoid taking over* unless it is absolutely necessary.

Depression

One of the worrying and increasingly common features of response to stress in modern times is depression. Research indicates that it is common amongst people with long-term illness, especially people with cancer. You may find that the person you care for is anxious and depressed. Look out for these classic signs of clinical depression:

- lack of appetite and weight loss, constipation
- lack of interest in sex and activity in general
- listlessness, always complaining of feeling tired and lethargic
- low mood, undue pessimism, lack of self-confidence, agitated and emotional lability, fluctuating emotions, crying then elation
- poor concentration, unable to read a book or hold a conversation for long
- sleep disturbance, cannot get off to sleep, early-morning waking
- waking up feeling tired and lacking in energy
- preoccupation with morbid thoughts and negativity
- in some cases, talking about suicide and having desperate thoughts.

(adapted from Rose 1988).

The list is not comprehensive and includes some of the things found in normal so-called healthy people.

Shirley Trickett (2001), herself a nurse, has written that people with depression often complain that they have no interest in anyone or anything. They commonly complain that *they know they still love their family, but they cannot feel it.* There are many types of depression – for example, mixed depression associated with dealing with difficult life circumstances and a feeling of being unable to cope with stimulus from inside the person as well as outward signs such as poor relationships at work. In other cases, agitated depression is seen when the person is restless, low in mood, but it's almost as if the person is unable to rest and be lethargic, like others with depression do. It is not always easy to observe that someone has depression, especially when you think that some people may deserve to feel fed up because of their life situation. An example of a complex and unusual problem that is not often seen in the UK is Chronic Fatigue Syndrome (CFS), which is a long-term illness or syndrome characterized by constant, overwhelming fatigue, lymphadenopathy (inflammation of the lymph glands), headache, myalgia, arthralgia and memory loss. People with CFS suffer from immunological and neurological impairment and may experience a range of vague viral-type illnesses. Some CFS patients have been known to suffer from exactly the same immune system problems as AIDS patients. American physicians have been studying the relationship between CFS and AIDS to examine if there is a link between the two conditions. Current results are inconclusive.

We may all experience low moods from time to time – for example, following bereavement or during a personal crisis. Treatment of depression does not necessarily involve taking prescribed medication and can involve sensitive, supportive listening, information giving, counselling and the use of a range of complementary therapies and herbal medicines such as St John's Wort. In some cases prescribed medication in the form of anti-depressants can be used alongside drugs to help with sleep problems or mild sedatives to alleviate anxiety symptoms. The GP is the key person to seek help and advice from. Taking medication should supplement good social support that uses active listening as a way of making sure that concerns and worries are shared and dealt with as and when they arise. As a concluding thought, anxiety and depression are not exclusive to people with long-term illness and many carers experience psychological difficulties in carrying out their carer role. Being self-aware can prevent difficulties becoming problems for the carer as well as the patient.

Communication and confusion

One of the biggest challenges facing carers occurs when the patient is confused or has difficulties in communication. This can include people with conditions such as strokes (right-sided), cerebral palsy, mental impairment disorders and late-stage Motor Neurone Disease. Communication problems can give rise to frustration for carers and patients and in some instances this can lead to them both becoming depressed and experiencing anxiety. Getting to know the person and becoming familiar with their problems, moods and needs can help tremendously. Speech difficulties (for example, only having a very limited vocabulary) can challenge, but they can be overcome. I recall an elderly gentleman (Harry) who had a severe stroke affecting his right side and speech centre in his brain. He could only say the word 'no', and this was the sum total of his vocabulary. At first it was a nightmare for us both, as he became frustrated at me (and vice versa). Other people, like his wife, knew how his tone of voice changed and had different meanings according to his needs. Speaking and saying 'no' slowly meant 'no', whereas increased and repetitive 'nos' meant 'yes'. Confusing? Yes it was, but after a while a sense of logic emerged. What really helped was that Harry could read; we had a communication board to hand all the time. He could also use drawings and write on pieces of paper and whiteboards, with symbols on to supplement communication. More contemporary forms of communication aids use computerized equipment that enhances communication greatly and provides simulated forms of digitalized speech, but also requires a good working knowledge. Most computerized equipment has made a fantastic change to communication ability, although when caring for people with speech difficulties it is vital to always have paper (card) and pen (marker) available in case of machine failure! Electronic communication boards can be enhanced and customized to incorporate useful and frequently used symbols that are specific to the patient and carer.

Rules of thumb – verbal problems

- Greet with a smile.
- Sit and face the patient and be at their level.
- Improve your non-verbal communication, smile a lot and use facial muscles.
- Open your mouth fully.
- Use appropriate touch to help convey meaning.
- Learn to read the patient's gestures.

- Learn to speak clearly and slowly (ask a speech and language therapist for help).
- Avoid complex questions.
- Customize communication – close eyes means 'yes', squeeze hand means 'no'.

Above all, try to anticipate your patient's needs and prepare in advance. For example, when helping them to get dressed if you know what the patient needs in advance, this avoids much frustration and improves communication. It is useful to ensure electronic aids such as possums are set up properly, understood by both parties and regularly serviced (remember back-up battery facilities).

Sources of specialist help

Speech and language therapists, occupational therapists and physiotherapists are useful people to help with practical communication issues. Speech and language therapists are very useful in helping patients to develop speech patterns and (re-)learn to swallow and breathe effectively. These days, technicians for electronic communication devices are also good to have on hand.

Helping someone who is confused

The term 'confusion' is often used by nursing and medical staff to refer to a patient's inability to understand what is going on around them. Whether the cause of the confusion is due to dehydration in an older person (toxic confusional state), circulatory problems (atherosclerosis) or an organic brain disorder such as dementia, the outcome often causes anxiety for the patient and carer alike. Remember that not all confusion is permanent (toxic confusion is easily remedied by increased fluids). Carers face a huge challenge to meet the patient's needs and to be able to communicate effectively. Sometimes it is not possible to have a coherent conversation or dialogue that others are able to follow. Often it is necessary to anticipate need and try to think in advance about what the patient is trying to tell you based on previous experience and personal knowledge. Wanting to go to the toilet is an obvious need after a drink or a meal. Often basic requirements to stand up, walk or stretch can create their own confusion. On a more psychological note, trying to understand a person who is very confused requires tact, patience and a generous spirit. It is all too easy to adopt a patronizing tone and humour the patient. Many have asked me whether it's okay to pretend or 'humour' patients when you have no idea what the context of the conversation is. Much depends on intent. For some carers and patients, it is important that a response is made, so that a degree of normality can take place. The type of response depends on the carer's attitude. Acknowledging the patient, and responding appropriately and sincerely need not be viewed as humouring them, but rather as learning to try and be with them and understand what their confusion is about and how it affects them. Sometimes severely confused people can suddenly become quite upset and tearful. Being prepared for this and responding with empathy can communicate what we ourselves would want to happen.

What can friends and family do?

- A key issue relating to carers' attitudes to confused patients is to consider how we might like to be treated if the roles were reversed.
- The essence of communicating with people with advanced dementia is to reflect on the qualities of the carer in Chapter 1: respect for the person, empathy with their situation, compassion and understanding in our thoughts, words and deeds.
- Become familiar with the effects and side effects of medication.
- Be aware that mood changes can be rapid, and try not to feel that some statements made by the patient are personal attacks.

- Remember the importance of rest for both the patient and the carer!
- Try to get help and have breaks from your caring role.

With long-term illness, confusion can often become more advanced as the patient's condition deteriorates. When this occurs, it is important to provide the care required to ensure that their dignity and respect remain as intact as possible.

Preventing carer burnout

Caring for a person who is confused can be very frustrating for the carer. The constant repetition – 'When are we going out?' 'Is Mary coming soon?' – can cause carers to become exasperated, especially if they are physically unwell, tired or just feeling stressed! The increased incidence of abuse in older people by carers is an indication of how difficult and frustrating it can become when caring for a person who is not able to remember what day it is, the time or (often) who you are. Buijssen (2005) points out that many nurses find it difficult to cope with very demanding patients, who are often confused and may be terminally ill. She uses the term 'burnout' to depict a situation where the carer experiences stress to a point where he or she can no longer maintain their normal professional self. Others discuss compassion fatigue whereby carers run out of empathy and compassion and find it hard to respond positively. What can be done to counter these distressing experiences?

There are several ways we can all improve our way of coping with difficulties when caring for others:

- Take time out and include periods of rest in your day.
- Ensure you get a good night's sleep or take a nap during the day.
- Make sure that if caring for a confused person there is some respite care planned to take the care burden away from you (see Chapter 7 for more details).

- Make sure you take exercise – even just a short walk – every day.
- Stay healthy, have a well-balanced diet and take plenty of water every day.
- Talk about your caring role, even if it is for a short period at the end of the day, or get to know someone in a professional carer's role who will offer support (see Chapter 7, p. 123).
- Avoid long periods when you are responsible for the patient alone.
- Do not allow yourself to become physically tired to the point where you cannot manage all the situations you are responsible for.

Being a carer is an important responsibility. To carry out this role effectively, carers need to be physically and mentally fit, as well as being supported themselves. Without this support, carers risk being unable to make the types of decisions they are required to and if physically worn out their judgments can become impaired and they may feel things are getting on top of them. Professional care providers in hospital and other settings have support strategies in place to avoid burnout. This is an important issue. Carers need to prevent the situation getting out of hand and to avoid finding ourselves in a stressful situation. Once they suffer fatigue stress and burnout, it can have an adverse effect on physical and mental well-being and make them unable to function properly. Therefore it is important that all carers are aware of the signs of burnout and avoid getting into the situation in the first place.

Case study: Helen

Helen (29) was the main carer for her mother (Edna, aged 77), who had advanced Alzheimer's disease. Helen was divorced with no children and had moved back into the family home mainly because her mum had deteriorated, and her dad had died two years ago, just after Helen separated from her husband. At first, Helen combined looking after her mum with working at the local supermarket 22 hours a week. When she was not with her, the neighbour Gillian kept an eye on her mum, who was better then. One day her mum got out of the house and walked down the road looking for the cat (who had died 10 years ago). She was very nearly knocked down by a car and the police were called. Gillian was very upset and said she could not take on the responsibility of looking after Edna. Helen gave up her job and looked after her mum full-time. Helen found it hard, especially at night when her mum woke at 3.00 a.m. and wanted to make the fire and cook a fried breakfast. Physically her mum was quite active, but mentally her condition deteriorated over months and Helen became very frustrated and felt trapped. One night Edna woke at 3.30 a.m. and was trying to get out of the house, banging on the front door. Helen was so tired she slept through the noise and was woken by the police, who broke down the front door. Her mum was crying and the police thought she was alone in the house. Helen felt very guilty and ashamed of herself. The police called a social worker, who spent time with Helen listening to what she had been through lately with her mum, who seemed to recover from the trauma very quickly and went back to bed. Helen was relieved to have someone to talk to, but most of all for someone to listen to her for a change. It made such a difference. The social worker arranged respite care for a week and Edna went into a care home for a week. Helen went to visit some friends in Liverpool she had not seen in months. She was also able to go out for a drink and stayed out till 2.00 a.m. On Sunday she stayed in bed until lunchtime, watched TV and chilled out like she had wanted to, but had not been able to. By the time she picked her mum up, she felt physically and mentally fitter and more able to manage her. What made a difference was someone helping her and advising her about the best way to cope. Now she has regular weekly respite from Crossroads care scheme and is able to go out, be herself and care for her own needs.

Helen's story – whilst sad – is not unusual. It is important to realize that often carers care because they love the person they are caring for, or in some cases there is a sense that they feel obliged to become the main carer because there is no one else available or willing to take the role on. Whatever the circumstances, it is important that carers see their role as important and one that requires support and guidance. Few carers can provide quality care on their own. It is important to seek help and support, even if it amounts to being able to spend time doing the things you want to do. Having support means that you are often more able to give better care because you feel better about yourself. Consider the summary below, which highlights some of the key signs of burnout.

Signs of burnout

- constantly feeling physically tired and worn out
- feeling worried, insecure and indecisive
- poor sleeping habits, waking early or having problems getting to sleep
- irritable and short-tempered, snappy and lacking in tolerance
- difficulty in relaxing, lacking in concentration
- tendency to consume more alcohol and use recreational drugs
- lacking self-confidence, fed up and generally low in mood

Recognizing signs of deterioration

Caring for someone with a long-term illness involves being able to notice changes and make observations about the patient that others may not be aware of – for example, changes in physical ability or subtle changes in behaviour, mood or attitude. Because carers spend more time in intimate contact with the patient, it is possible for them to notice these small changes. It is necessary to become aware when the patient's physical and mental status changes or deteriorates. I have discussed signs of low mood and depression and how mood changes or grumpiness can be due to simple things like bowel problems (see Chapter 4). Likewise, an inability to walk unaided may be due to a fall, not seen by the carer. More symptomatic signs of ageing or the development of early onset dementia can be more difficult to identify, partly because the patient relies on the carer as their eyes and sometimes doing their thinking for them. 'Dementia' is a collective term for a disorder, that usually occurs in older people over the age of 65, although there are a tiny number of people affected under 65. It is not an inevitable cause of getting older. Dementia develops very gradually and is chiefly characterized by changes in disturbances of memory. Of all people suffering from dementia, roughly 55 per cent have Alzheimer's disease, a specific form of dementia. In other cases 15 per cent of people have vascular dementia, of which Multi-Infarct Dementia (MID) is well-known. In this case, damage to the blood supply causes oxygen loss to parts of the brain, causing tissue erosion. In many cases of early onset dementia, there is an inability to realize what you have just been doing, or forget what you are saying, or fail to recall relatively simple things like where the kettle is kept. In some cases, as Buijssen (2005) points out, it is like *the person finds themselves in a fog.* In many cases early onset dementia can be managed by putting it down to being forgetful. They can make excuses or make up a story to fit the lapse in memory confabulation. Carers need to be aware of these small changes, which at first may not seem to bother the patient until it becomes more obvious and harder to avoid. The carer's response should be a sensitive one. Often patients are aware of their own shortcomings and feel guilty, depressed and upset. They need support, but also guidance and reassurance. The carer needs to be aware that the patient may need greater supervision, and attention to the likelihood of safety issues, such as using the stove, lighting the gas fire and leaving doors unlocked. Specific problems can occur at night due to waking early, for example in Helen's story.

Early signs of dementia

- becoming forgetful; forgetting where everyday articles go
- putting things in the wrong place, for example, teabags in the fridge
- lack of memory for the recent past, such as the morning or day before, although memory for past events seems to remain intact
- lack of concentration; inability to read for periods of time
- a vague sense of restlessness and distraction

What can friends and family do?

Friends and family can and do play an important part in supporting people with early onset dementia. Remaining sensitive to changes in mood and behaviour is important, as is not paying too much attention to minor memory lapses. Learn to communicate effectively and avoid patronizing behaviour or reinforcing inappropriate behaviour (see earlier in this chapter). It is important to seek advice and help. The GP is a good source and they may refer you to a specialist in psychological medicine, often a psychiatrist. In some cases, the gradual onset of the condition means that the person can be cared for in their own home for a long time. Change, in terms of moving to a home, even for respite, can be stressful, although people with dementia do adapt to new environments with skilled help and support from professional staff and family and friends.

Summary

This chapter has focused on psychological issues. Often these are the most challenging to manage, and the most difficult problems to come to terms with, as there are often no easy answers. Confused patients and those with dementia need time, patience and understanding to enable others to accept changes in the person, often someone they have known all their life, a person they love and someone they have relied on earlier in life. Observing someone change is a very difficult situation to deal with. Communicating effectively when someone has psychological problems can, and *does*, make a difference. Whether the person is depressed, losing their ability to self-manage or becoming forgetful, active listening is the carer's key skill. The patient will benefit from having someone they can turn to, talk to and be comforted by. Being able to listen well, respond empathically and show concern, through responding to their emotions, can make a lot of difference to a person. The carer is ideally placed to emotionally engage with the patient, learn to understand their needs and observe changes in their behaviour. In some cases, this can prove to be invaluable in identifying and responding to changes indicative of some other pathology. More than anything, this chapter has highlighted the need for carers to be aware of their own well-being and to accept the need for support to avoid developing burnout. Physically, carers are able to provide important support. The quality of their care is also dependent on their ability to stay physically and mentally strong.

6

Care at the end of life

Caring for a person who has had a long-term illness at the end of their life can be both challenging and rewarding. Professional nurses often report that they feel privileged to have shared the last part of a person's life, as it is often a time when intimate moments can be shared and a great deal of satisfaction can be experienced by both the cared for and the care provider. At the same time, however, it needs to be stressed that end-of-life care can also be very difficult and distressing for all concerned. Carers make a difference throughout the time they spend caring for the patient. Towards the end of life, they have an impact and exert a positive influence on the dying person, enabling them and the family to experience a *good death*. A good death has been described as one where the patient and family not only have control over events at the end of life, but also are helped to exercise this control (Taylor 1993). Good deaths tend not to involve the patient experiencing pain and distress, and challenge those looking after the dying person, both professional and lay carers, to manage and control symptoms. The purpose of this chapter is to describe what carers can do to make a difference at the end of life and to help provide the patient and family with the least distressing and hopefully positive experience – a good death. The chapter begins by looking at attitudes towards death and the importance of good communication. It will include ways of managing physical symptoms that may arise in the latter stages of life and the types of psychological care that are an essential part of what many call terminal care. Essentially the chapter considers two distinct types of approach to end-of-life care; good and bad deaths – contrasting how the carer can often (but not always) influence and enable the patient and the family to experience death with sadness but not regret.

Attitudes towards death

We are all going to die and death is one of the few irreducible facts of life. However, there are differing views on whether there is a stigma about death in the UK. Some authors argue that death is stigmatized and attitudes towards it indicate that, as a subject, it is often ignored (Copp 1999). Others argue that in the last decade or more there has been a growing interest or revival of interest in death (Walters 1994). Despite the debates, it is clear that people vary in their views towards death, and as a subject it is not the number one topic of conversation in most households. Attitudes toward death and dying are important for all carers, because they have a responsibility for supporting dying people at the end of life. Often death threatens our sense of mortality and can make us afraid to discuss it with patients and families. In other cases, our personal experience can often prejudice our attitude and perhaps cause us to think that one person's loss is much the same as another. Having experienced personal loss, however, is no guarantee that we will be qualified (and able) to help others, but it may make us slightly more sensitive to the needs of others. One of the key issues in caring for a dying person is good communication from the time of diagnosis up until, and after, the death itself.

Communication about dying

One of the key communication issues focuses on a question people often ask, and one that doctors are often unable to answer accurately: 'How long have I got before I die?' This is the big question. The reason doctors cannot answer this question truthfully is because they do not know. At the same time it is unwise to speculate and be insensitive, since many people would place emphasis on this type of information. Doctors are often likely to say things such as 'How long is a piece of string' and state fairly that they do not know for sure. Patients and families who push for more detail, such as an indication of months or weeks 'to go', may find that the doctor is willing to make a bold statement if they think the prognosis is fairly clear. However, more often the prognosis is unclear and much depends on the patient's physical condition at the time.

There is an argument for people with life-limiting illness *not* being made aware of the whole truth about the diagnosis as this can cause unnecessary distress (Costello 2006). Conversely, some families prefer to know as much as possible about the diagnosis, illness, prognosis and what is referred to as dying trajectory (the period when the person is facing impending death). Because dying is such a difficult subject for most people, there is often a fear of knowing, and at the same time a desire to be told what to expect. Often people rely on doctors and nurses to tell them what to do, so they can start to prepare and make the necessary adjustments to their lives. Being told that you have a life-threatening medical illness that is likely to end your life in the near future is something that alters a person's outlook on life from that moment onwards. Carers need to be aware of the profound changes that can take place.

Providing terminal care

'Terminal care' is the term used when caring for a person at the end of their life. It is related to (but distinct from) palliative care, which refers to care from the moment of diagnosis up to and including death. Good terminal care includes many of the issues previously discussed in this book, placing emphasis on preventing problems, reducing distress and promoting psychological well-being. This includes making sure that those close to the patient are as involved in the care as possible, irrespective of the context in which dying takes place. In the home setting it is important that care is based on a team approach. This will invariably include the community nurses as well as the Macmillan nurse, if appropriate. Good care includes meeting the patient's physical and psychological needs. These can include:

- physical well-being, feeling clean and well cared for
- feeling well nourished and hydrated
- meeting the patient's elimination needs for going to the toilet
- controlling pain and other symptoms
- maintaining psychological well-being.

Physical well-being in the home can be achieved with help from others. Carers should not be reluctant to use professional help at all times. The key issue is coordination. Community nurses work around the clock, although the majority are available 9 to 5. It is useful to try and establish a pattern whereby the community nurse is able to contribute when required – for example, helping the patient get out of bed, washed and dressed. Nursing procedures can be carried out, such as dressings, catheter care, care, and injections. Pain control can also be given (prior to activity) and the patient assessed and monitored for changes, be it deterioration or improvement. Preventing complications such as pressure sores is vital, as this may add to pain and discomfort. The use of special pressure-relieving mattresses and seats (when in the chair) to provide comfort can alleviate discomfort and prevent soreness developing. Regular movement is essential. If the patient needs to be in bed, regular turning (at least every two hours is required) may be a key task.

When considering a strategy for providing physical care, it is useful to think about doing many things at once, such as moving the patient, using the toilet, relieving pressure, having a drink or eating while help is available and to prevent the patient being disturbed. Despite being ill, the patient also needs rest and comfort. Ensuring the involvement of community nurses at the right time is invaluable, especially if they can be flexible and attend when you need them to.

Providing good pain and symptom relief is a key issue. Being able to prevent pain is a challenge. Giving pain relief before movement or activity will ensure that the patient is kept pain-free and anticipates that pain may occur at certain times. At the same time, it may be necessary to include anti-sickness medication with the pain relief. Pain can also be relieved by more simple means, such as changing the patient's position, standing them up, distraction, engaging them in conversation, offering massage and using music or television. During office hours care provision may seem easy compared to providing care at night or after 5.00 p.m. when resources are more scarce. This is where it becomes necessary to develop good relations with the community nurses (having mobile phone numbers and GP contact numbers). Having a syringe driver (a portable device enabling a hypodermic syringe to give drugs slowly over a long time period) to provide pain relief is an excellent system, but the syringe does need to be changed (often every 12 hours) with medication prescribed and given to prevent breakthrough pain.

What about the carer?

Providing good terminal care is very hard work and the care provider is at their most vulnerable at this time. The key to providing quality care is often coordination and anticipation. This involves using other people to relieve you as the main carer and for you to have rest and time to yourself. There is a lot to think about and prepare for. Sleep and rest are important for both you and the patient. It is necessary for you to plan relief and to delegate. Ask others to step in and take over the role of carer to enable you to get out, take fresh air, go to the cinema, have a drink, visit a friend or go to the park for a walk. To do these things often requires some form of structure or routine. This is not a bad thing, as others will know what is happening and what their role is. Routines help people carry out their tasks and plan for the future. Include the patient as much as possible, but planning to include flexibility is key. Consider asking the community nurse to try and come on demand, rather than at the same time each day. Also, if the Macmillan nurse is involved, see if they can come for an hour and be with the patient while you go out. Can other family members or friends patient sit for periods of time on request? Helping you as the carer is directly linked with helping the patient.

Anticipatory grief

In general terms most people in the UK are made aware that they have a terminal illness, even though when they are first diagnosed the full extent of their disease may not be made clear. When faced with impending death, people react differently. There are a number of ways people respond to hearing that they have a life-threatening medical illness (Kubler-Ross 1991):

- anger and shock
- denial ('It can't be – it's a mistake')
- bargaining ('What happens if I stop smoking/take more exercise/get better/ lose weight?')
- depression (resign themselves negatively to the fact of death and become fed up depressed and uncooperative)
- acceptance (accept their fate – 'We all have to go at some time')

The impact of bad news varies with individuals. Some people may accept the news at once; others may go through the above stages, even in order; while others may become depressed and then angry. There is no *one way* that people react to hearing that they have a limited amount of time left to live. There is, in other words, no chronology to dying. The famous American comedian Lenny Bruce, considering the above stages, quipped that he would skip the first four and go straight to acceptance, as it seems less painful.

It is important to develop and maintain a sense of hope when hearing the bad news. Kubler-Ross (1991) felt that it was essential for doctors and nurses to acknowledge the importance of having a sense of hope about the future. Death could be a long way off and having a sense of purpose, expectation and a positive outlook is important in order to maintain well-being and have something to look forward to. In this way the phrase 'Take one day at a time' has particular meaning. For carers who may also be relatives or emotionally close to the patient, it can be very difficult to adapt to the impending loss. For both the patient and the carers, this adjustment may be experienced as a sense of anticipatory grief (Costello 1997). This experience, unlike the conventional understanding of grief, which begins after death, is different in many ways. Anticipatory grief considers that the emotions involved in losing another person begin to take place from the time the person is diagnosed and stops at the time of death. During this time, *both* the patient and carer/family members can experience the emotional impact that occurs when someone is dying. It is also possible to adapt to the new situation when the patient is going to die. This can involve a number of things, from talking about the death, making a will, discussing funeral plans and making wishes about death known to others. This sounds very organized and practical, but in reality is very painful, emotional and an extremely difficult time for carers. This is why some people prefer not to think about it and deny the existence of a diagnosis, despite being told the bad news. As carers, it is important not only to understand the patient's reaction, but also to respect that this is the way they feel. It may alter and change over time. Some people on hearing the bad news may wish to remain in denial. They may find it too difficult to talk about or organize. Some may annoy others because they want to organize, discuss, plan and prepare by making a funeral plan and organizing the service. The key issues regarding anticipatory grief are that they allow the following to take place:

- discussion about dying
- planning and preparation for death to take place
- spiritual care to be provided
- grief to be openly expressed
- wishes and desires to be made known
- grief to be shared between the carer/family/friends and the patient.

Making a will

Good end-of-life care includes making a number of preparations including writing a will. A will is a written legal document prepared by the patient (the 'testator'), that sets out what will happen to their property, assets and wealth less any outstanding liabilities (your 'estate') when they die. The will includes provisions for appointing a guardian for any children under the age of 18 the patient may have. The will also appoints one or more executors, who carry out the instructions in the will. As a carer, in some cases unbeknown to you, you may also become an executor of the patient's will.

Having a will ensures that the patient's estate is dealt with according to their wishes. Without a will your assets may end up being distributed by prescribed regulations 'intestacy laws'. It is not the case, as many assume, that if a husband or wife dies their estate automatically passes to their spouse. A substantial amount may go to other relatives.

A will ensures that the patient's estate is distributed as they would like it to be, and that loved ones are properly provided for. It will also ensure the people you give your estate to do not have to pay more tax than necessary. A will document can be purchased at a stationery outlet or be professionally drawn up by a solicitor for a fee. Witnesses need to sign the will in the presence of the person making the will and it needs to be kept safe and, if necessary, amended and witnessed again if circumstances or wishes change.

Making advance decisions at the end of life (living wills)

In contemporary society, as a result of a range of issues (many of which originate from the Human Rights Act 2005), individuals are increasingly being empowered to make decisions about how they wish to be treated in terms of health, education and death. Towards the end of life people are making what are called advanced decisions or statements (previously 'living wills') pertaining to their wishes – chiefly a refusal to have life-sustaining treatments. Advanced decisions/statements are legally enforceable documents (see p. 102), usually written at or towards the end of life, that relate to the patient's wishes when their condition becomes terminal. Often advanced statements of this kind are made when the patient wishes to stipulate their right to refuse treatment. Requests for certain types of treatment such as transplants and investigations, however, are not legally binding, whereas advanced statements provide for a better understanding of how patients would like to be treated. Carers may wish to consider the patient's wishes and preferences and help them to formulate an advanced statement if the patient has specific things that they wish not happen to them – for example, a preference not to be tube-fed or not to be resuscitated in the event of cardiac arrest. Advanced statements enable people to make their own choices about their own lives, in accordance with their individual beliefs. If an advanced statement is not made, the family will not have any legal right to act on the patient's behalf regarding refusal of treatments. Advanced statements are recognized as legally binding documents by a number of organizations, including;

- Age Concern
- British Medical Association
- Royal College of Nursing
- General Medical Council
- Nursing and Midwifery Council
- Law Society

Advanced statements can be obtained from many sources. They can be written yourself or purchased commercially from many companies, such as Law Pack and the Voluntary Euthanasia Society. Some advanced statements can also be used to nominate a Health Care Proxy – for example, a carer, friend or relative – who knows your wishes and can communicate them to the medical team on your behalf. Advanced statements can only be used to accept or refuse legal medical treatment, not actively to end life.

Example of an advanced decision (also known as living will) document

ADVANCED DECISION

TO MY FAMILY, MY DOCTOR AND ALL CONCERNED.

This Advanced Decision is made by me:
I am fully aware that I have .... and that it is a progressive, degenerative condition for which there is no cure.

At a time when I am of sound mind and after careful consideration, I DECLARE that if at any time the following circumstances exist, namely:

1. I am unable to communicate effectively
2. I have become unable to participate effectively in decisions about my medical care, and
3. I am unlikely to recover from severe illness or impairment involving or expected to cause me severe distress or incapacity for rational existence.

Then, and in those circumstances, my directions are as follows:

1. That I am not to be subjected to the following medical interventions or treatments aimed at prolonging or sustaining my life:
   a) resuscitation in the event of cardiac arrest or sudden collapse and if such an arrest happens in my own home, I would not wish paramedics to be called
   b) any medication given by intravenous drips

c) any artificial feeding or hydration by any method
d) any antibiotics.

2. That any distressing symptoms (including any caused by lack of food or fluid) are to be fully controlled by appropriate palliative care, ordinary nursing care, analgesics and/or sedation, even though that treatment may shorten my life.

All of these directions are to be followed when my life is at risk, preferably enabling me to die at home.

I nominate my ...., ..., to be consulted by my medical attendants, when considering what my wishes and intentions would be in any uncertain situation.

I have talked this over with my general practitioner.

GP signature: ....
Name: ....
Telephone number: ....
GP Address: ....
....
....

Maker's signature: ....

WITNESS:
I testify that .... ,
the maker of this Directive, signed it in my presence and made it clear to me that he understood what it meant. I do not know of any pressure being brought on him to make such a Directive and I believe it was made by his own wish.

Witness Signature: ....
Name: ....
Telephone number: ....
Witness address: ....
....
....

What can friends and family do?

At the end of life, family and friends play a very important role in supporting the patient and in the experience of dying and death. Respecting the wishes of the patient is key to helping them feel that they have influence and control over what is happening. This can be very difficult at times, especially if the patient is in hospital. There are many decisions that need to be made at this time, not least of all where the patient prefers to receive care and eventually die. Most people, when asked for a preference, state that they would prefer to die at home (Seale & Kelly 1997), even though the majority of people die in hospital. Being involved in making choices about end-of-life care is important in terms of exercising control and eventually experiencing a good death. Government guidance on preferred place of care (Department of Health 2004) states that patients should be asked about their preferences, and wherever possible these should be adhered to. Some people may choose to die in hospital because it is a secure safe place and there is less of a burden on carers. Others may wish to die in a local hospice or at home. Dying at home surrounded by your family is an ideal, although often difficult for some people (Costello 1990). Families and friends can help the patient to come to a decision that helps them experience emotional support at the end of their life. Dying at home requires resources, support from professionals and family and a lot of determination. Older, frail, vulnerable people may find it hard to manage the death of a spouse at home, especially if they are suffering from illness themselves. Wanting to die in hospital is a sign that the patient wants security, although visiting and coping with hospital communication can be daunting. If end-of-life care is in hospital, it may be useful to consider some key issues:

- Ask for a side room if the patient/family would prefer more privacy.
- Ensure that staff are aware of spiritual needs – for example to request sacrament of the sick at the appropriate time.

● Discuss with hospital staff details regarding who to call and when to call family should the patient's condition deteriorate suddenly.

● Maintain communication at all times and know that you are able to make an appointment to see the consultant should you wish to discuss care or treatment with them.

● Make sure that any issues relating to living wills, such as requests not to actively intervene should the patient have a cardiac or respiratory arrest, are communicated directly to hospital staff as soon as possible on or after admission.

● Arrange financial support by enabling the patient to receive Attendance Allowance if they do not already receive this – under special rules (see Chapter 7, p. 128).

Support

Whether at home, in hospital or in a hospice, there are a number of sources of support at the end of life. Much of the support is charity based and one of the key charities is Macmillan Cancer Relief, a large UK-based charity who provide support, advice and financial help to people with cancer. Community nurses, social workers and other health care professionals can advise and make referrals to Macmillan nurses, who specialize in providing help at the end of life for cancer patients. There are also numerous non-cancer organizations and support groups who can provide help and support (see Chapter 7).

Spiritual care

Spirituality is a complex subject, often closely linked to religion, that relates to individual values and beliefs, and (when related to end of life care) focuses on the various meanings people give to their lives. When a person is facing impending death, it may be a source of comfort to make efforts to *close their lives* and begin to make efforts to come to terms with what their life has amounted to. For some, this is closely related to religious practice and carers may wish to seek advice from members of the clergy or a priest. For some Catholics, it is important that sacrament of the sick is given before death (at any point), in order to feel absolved from sin. Some people may *find their faith* when facing death and wish to discuss their religious views with a member of the hospital chaplaincy department or religious leader. For agnostics or atheists, it may be a question of seeking spiritual guidance from a humanist. Humanists claim to number 36 per cent of the population – about 17 million in total. They believe in self-determination of man without religious involvement. Humanists believe in spirituality but not in any form of religious practice. Many areas in the UK have a local Humanist branch that offers support to humanists at the end of life.

Saying goodbye

Practically and symbolically, it is important for everyone associated with the patient to say goodbye in their own way. This does not mean attending the place of death, the funeral or seeing them when they were dying. Often family and friends like to have opportunities to say their own goodbye around the time of the death. This can occur more easily when the person dies at home as there is no restriction to accessing the patient. If the patient dies in a hospital/hospice or nursing/care home, the staff invariably arrange a time for what is called 'viewing the deceased' prior to transfer to the chapel of rest. Once it becomes clear that the patient is close to death (and this can be very difficult to predict and know), if not already in attendance the family will be contacted and asked to come in. Family and close friends are able to view the patient before being transferred to the hospital mortuary or taken by the funeral director to the chapel of rest. This is one opportunity for family and friends to say goodbye. The family can also arrange for a member of the church or faith group to be present as well and an informal goodbye or prayer ritual can take place. Other such rituals can take place in the chapel of rest.

Practical issues at the end of life

Whether the death of the patient is expected or sudden, it is often a sad time and may cause shock for some. Family and friends may react differently at this time. Some may express a sense of relief that the patient has been taken out of their suffering and their death is seen as a blessing. Others may have hoped that the person would live long and put off the inevitable using denial – in which case, they may be shocked and very upset at the time of death. As previously discussed, it is not unusual to see expressions of anger, sadness, shock, disbelief and acceptance. As a carer it is useful to know about the actions taken by professionals at the time of death and to be able to explain these to others, who may feel too upset to appreciate what is taking place. In most cases, the professionals are aware of the sensitivity of the situation and will act appropriately. Where the death is expected and the GP or hospital doctor is aware of the cause of death, the events that take place at and around the time of death are predictable. Once death has been verified, a doctor needs to examine the patient and issue a death certificate, which enables a funeral director to take them to the chapel of rest.

Should the death be sudden, or where the circumstances of the death are unclear, it is necessary to hold an inquest to determine and investigate the exact cause of death. In some cases – for example, if the patient is admitted to hospital within 48 hours and dies suddenly and no clear diagnosis was established – it is necessary to conduct a postmortem. This is standard procedure in order to find out and record the accurate cause of death in any institution such as a hospital, hospice and nursing/care home. It will invariably always take place if the patient died as a result of an accident such as a road traffic accident. The purpose of the postmortem is to verify the exact cause of death.

The death certificate is issued once the postmortem has taken place. If the death was at home and anticipated, the GP will issue the death certificate having seen and confirmed their death. Since the Shipman case, however (where a Derbyshire GP was found guilty of killing elderly people at home using morphine), authorities are exercising extra vigilance in checking the circumstances of certain deaths at home. This includes older, vulnerable people who die at home, and the death is investigated often several weeks and months after the death and funeral have taken place. This is necessary but distressing for the grieving family. Any delay in managing the funeral is likely to cause further distress, especially if the cause of death was unclear. Family members and friends often feel a sense of guilt at the time of death and investigations tend to increase the sense of well-being that is associated with sudden death.

Grief and bereavement

As a carer you will experience a sense of loss at the death of the patient, who may also be a friend, spouse or sibling. You may also be in a position to provide support for the grieving family. It is useful to consider what bereavement support may entail and how you can support the family in this way after death.

Grief is complex and individual, although there seems to be some similarities in the way people express their feelings before and after death. Some express their feelings and talk about their emotions easily and sometimes excessively; others feel more secure in keeping their feelings to themselves. These are sometimes called feminine and masculine ways of grieving. It is important to distinguish between the two and avoid forcing those comfortable with their silence to open up and be able to listen to those who prefer to share their feelings. Offering support after death can take many forms. In the classic sense, you may offer people the opportunity to talk about their feelings and provide a listening ear, which is often an underrated and invaluable form of support. After death, the nature of our relationship with the deceased, as well as the circumstances of the death, cause us to reflect on the loss and in many ways rethink our future, often influencing our well-being. Active listening is an important way of helping someone feel understood and can help people make sense of the confusing and sometimes negative feelings experienced after death. Offering support after death can also involve practical help such as offering to visit the graveside, sharing a job that has been put off for many months or just being there for a person who finds loneliness hard to cope with. It need not involve becoming a mini counsellor as some people would not want this! The key issues are to do with helping the person through a difficult time and being observant for signs that the natural process of grief is not being followed.

Signs of grief becoming complicated

The majority of people in the UK who experience bereavement pass through this normal healthy process unscathed. Others may experience a profound sadness and require further help. As a carer it is useful to recognize the signs of grief becoming complicated. As a carer you may feel obliged to offer support to other friends and family. In doing so, it is useful to be aware that there are certain observations you may make that indicate that the person's grief is causing them great distress. There is no specific time limit to experiencing grief. It has been suggested that up to two years may pass before the person is able to fully engage in the things they want to, despite pangs of sadness about the loss for the rest of their lives (Parkes 1972). Much depends on the nature of the relationship with the deceased, how they died and the mourner's ability to cope. The key risk factors focus on whether there is previous psychiatry history (especially of depression), making it hard for the person to cope effectively. Some mourners find it hard to get over the death if it has been marred by tragedy (a bad death), where the patient was perceived to die in pain. This can lead to chronic grief reaction or a situation where the mourner blames themselves and the grief is exaggerated. It is important that, as a carer, you are not responsible for providing others with bereavement support after death. It is useful to be aware of your limitations and seek help from others if you feel that the mourner appears to be suffering excessively and not responding to support from others. The following signs (not one on its own) indicate that the person may develop difficulties and perhaps suggest a need for more professional support (see the useful contacts list for guidance).

- history of depression/ psychiatric treatment in the past
- limited social network, few friends and family members to offer support
- unemployment and lack of finances
- circumstances of the loss, sudden or traumatic (bad) death

Summary

This chapter has considered ways in which the carer can help to influence and shape the patient's end-of-life care to enable the patient and family to experience a good death. It is important that physical (terminal) care is of a very high standard, for obvious reasons, but also the standard of care influences the perceptions of those emotionally attached to the patient, including the carer. It is also important to consider that, for many, irrespective of their relationship to the patient, grieving begins from the time the diagnosis is made and awareness of dying takes place. Family members and friends may begin to adapt to the impending loss and some may not demonstrate their grief in textbook fashion. This may be due to having experienced anticipatory grief during the (sometimes long) process of the illness. Care at the end of life includes both practical help such as making a will and caring for the spirit. This is a major challenge for anyone. The carer may have been providing support for months and years and is called up to produce some of the best care at a time when the patient is dying. This can cause worry, distress and physical exhaustion. The carer is more vulnerable to stress and burn out at this time more than any other. Moreover, the carer may be called upon to provide support to others *after death* and to be aware that people react in many ways to loss. Sometimes the grief can become complicated and knowing what to look for can help to reduce the distress often experienced after the loss of loved one. A good death can be looked back on with sadness but within a sense of satisfaction that the person was loved, cared for and missed without too much regret.

7

Getting help and support for the patient and the carer

Introduction

One of the key themes of this book has been promoting the patient's well-being. Closely aligned with this is the well-being of the carer, who is a highly valued part of the care provided to the person with a long-term illness. This chapter will include suggestions and guidance on how friends and family members can help the carer in terms of providing support and respite. An important part of the carer's coping strategies includes taking a break from caring and having a support structure available to help maintain and develop their sense of well-being. The purpose of this chapter is to identify and describe sources of help for carers and explain how to access these important resources. It begins by considering how to make the caring environment (often the home) a safe and secure setting. The chapter also identifies some well-known support groups, such as Crossroads care schemes, which improve the quality of care for the patient as well as enable the carer to discuss forms of self-help and strategies for enabling them to develop and maintain their own well-being. Being an effective carer means being able to look after yourself and staying healthy, both physically and psychologically. Being able to fulfil your role effectively means being aware, informed and supported at all times.

Safety in the home

An important part of any caring situation is the safety and security of those involved. In the home environment it is important to know that the carer and patient are safe and secure as this provides peace of mind. Practical services exist to ensure this. One such example is the local fire service, who provide free safety checks as well as a free smoke alarm and safety advice about a range of issues related to preventing fires in the home. The police will provide a similar service on home protection and offer advice on a range of security issues, from burglar alarms to safety chains on doors and protocols for admitting callers into the house. A telephone call to the local police and fire services will make sure this type of safety issue is dealt with. For carers who have specific needs in relation to their physical health, social services occupational therapists are able to provide a home assessment to advise on issues relating to the patient's ability to carry out Activities of Daily Living. They may point out floor coverings that are likely to cause falls (such as rugs and mats on slippery surfaces), and give advice on the installation of grab rails and ramps for wheel-chair users, as well as raised toilet seats, hoists and stair lifts. Be aware that local authorities differ in the services they provide. They also charge for adaptations, many of which are means-tested (although the advice is free). For patients with specific conditions such as MND, MS and Parkinson's disease, services and advice can also be obtained from the national associations (listed in the Resources section of this book). Practical help in doing any of the 101 jobs around the house can be obtained from a variety of sources, although it is often worthwhile seeking advice from professionals about what services are provided by local authorities and what specialist help can be obtained. The provision of these services makes the carer's life as well as that of the patient a lot less stressful.

Community nursing support

Statutory services like community nurses (also known as district nurses) are an invaluable source of support and advice. Community nurses are able to access primary care (community GP services) to help provide the patient receiving care at home with a range of services – for example, enabling them to borrow a NHS bed if necessary, or helping with aids such as commodes. They are also able to help with referral to other services, such as the continence advisor, for help with urinary problems, and other specialist nurses such as stoma nurses and Macmillan nurses. Community nurses are a direct link with GPs and often provide nursing care on behalf of the GP for older people in the community as well as those with established medical conditions. The community nursing service consists of qualified nurses who carry out a range of procedures – from giving insulin to diabetic patients to dressing wounds following discharge from hospital. The service includes unqualified assistant nurses, who support qualified nurses in providing nursing care for patients in their own home, and in care and nursing homes. Many also offer services that enable patients to attend the local hospital to receive treatment for established problems such as leg ulcers. The GP can make a referral for a visit from the community nurse. Social workers, occupational therapists, physiotherapists and other community-based staff can also make referrals. The patient or carer is advised to seek help via their GP, who will ask the nurse to visit often following a period in hospital. The nurse will conduct an assessment or provide direct hands-on care.

Caring for someone whilst working

Many carers combine their caring role with full- and part-time work. This can be very demanding and stressful. In some cases, you may be working when you start your caring role. When this happens, it is useful to tell your employer about your situation. There are several things you also need to consider. These will help you and the person being cared for when seeking effective services.

- Inform your employer, as you could be helped to work from home or have flexible working hours arranged.
- You could have your working hours altered or compressed. This is where you work your normal hours in a shorter period of time, typically fitting a five-day week into four days.
- Change to term time or annualized working hours (the number of hours you are contracted for per month or year is worked in a flexible way).
- You can develop a job share or change to part-time working.
- Holidays can be arranged to allow you to fit in your alternative care arrangements.

Changes in allowances regarding employment whilst caring are taking place all the time. From 2008, new flexible working time regulations will include unpaid (adult) carers being given the right (in addition to current parent carers) to request flexible working. This does not mean that they will automatically be given flexible working arrangements when they start. For further information see www.direct.gov.uk.

Emergency leave

Carers are entitled to emergency leave (whether paid or unpaid), but there are other leave arrangements that may be available, such as:

- carer's leave (paid or unpaid)
- borrowing or buying leave time
- compassionate leave
- career breaks.

If you have worked for your employer for more than a year, your employer is required to ensure that you receive reasonable time off to fulfil your caring commitments, especially if there is an emergency or other special circumstances you need to attend to. These can include:

- problems or a breakdown in planned care arrangements
- an episode of acute illness in the person being cared for
- if you need to attend care planning meetings or make arrangements for long-term care
- if your child has an accident at school
- if you need to take compassionate leave before or after the death of a dependent.

Support for the carer: working and caring

Many carers combine their role as carer with working on a part-time basis. The provision of certain statutory rights enables carers to fulfil their dual role of carer and worker. If you are a care provider for a member of your family or a friend, you can (for example) be granted carer's leave when your work commitments clash with your role as carer. In the past people in this position would claim personal sickness time if they were unable to attend work because the person they cared for was sick and required help at home. Section 1 of the Chronically Sick and Disabled Persons Act 1970 imposes a duty on the county council to find out the number of people who require services and to publish information about available services. It also gives people the right to complain to the Secretary of State for Health if they feel their local authority has not fulfilled its duty towards them.

The local authority is obliged to provide many areas of help, including:

- practical help in the home, radio and/or television and help to use the local library
- help to take advantage of educational facilities (including transport)
- adaptations or special equipment needs in the home to help with convenience or for safety
- holidays, meals and telephone (and special equipment to use it if needed).

Any provision of resources is dependent upon an assessment of need under the Chronically Sick and Disabled Persons Act 1970. The provisions of the Act remain in addition to the NHS and Community Care Act 1990. For more information, contact your local Disability Service.

The aim of the NHS and Community Care Act 1990 is to help people live safely in the community. Social services assess the needs of people and arrange for the provision of social care services to meet these needs. Other responsibilities include procedures for receiving comments and complaints, registration and inspection procedures, and the individual's ability to contribute.

For further help, view the NHS and Community Care Act website (see 'Resources and useful contacts' at the end of the book).

Understanding anxiety

Everyone experiences anxiety at some point in their lives depending on the type and amount of stress we encounter. As carers put themselves in a situation where it is likely they may experience stress as a result of their role, coping with stress seems like a useful and important thing to consider. This section looks at ways to help you to manage some of the anxiety and stress that can be (but not necessarily *is*) a part of being a carer.

We all manage stress differently. Some of us cry, others get angry or deny our feelings, others feel overwhelmed by our emotions and internalize our thoughts, refusing to (or feeling unable to) share them with others. As a result the worry and anxiety can become too difficult to deal with. Anxiety is worry or fear about what may happen as a result of things we may not be able to control – for example, worrying about a visit to the doctor, waiting for results from a medical check-up, being out of a job, having no money, feeling unpopular or having no friends, or not having a sense of security. Is it normal to feel anxious? In a sense yes, if you are the sort of person who is sensitive to what is happening to you and if you are in touch with your feelings. Some people are anxious but do not become aware of it as it manifests itself in different ways, such as feeling tired, ill or fed up. In some cases we may experience what is referred to as free-floating anxiety (Trickett 2001), which is a vague feeling of fear without knowing what may be causing it, and despite rationalising it by saying 'I am well, I am intelligent, have a lovely partner, no money problems, but I still feel anxious'.

What to do about anxiety

There are several ways of tackling anxiety. Much depends on the cause and how you deal with problems. Here are a few practical sound-bite approaches that may work for you.

- Talk things through with a friend, family member or colleague.
- Distract yourself by becoming engaged in a hobby.
- Keep fit or get fit – exercise is a great stress-buster.
- Join a group, educational or social, to share your experiences.
- Seek professional help.

Some or all of these things may appeal to you. A popular phrase these days is 'It's good to talk'. The resolution of many psychological problems is based on the talking therapies. Talking things through, sharing your feelings and giving vent to your emotions is designed to help you see them in perspective, to put them in a better light. Often there is no cure as such, but talking things over with a trusted person or a stranger can help you to see things in a different light. A bad listener may give you their experiences instead and you may think that, compared to your problems, theirs are worse! Not everyone finds it easy to share their feelings, especially if they are not sure what these are! Talking to no one is hard – talking to someone can be harder still. A popular form of professional help these days is cognitive behavioural therapy (CBT). This centres around the idea that you can influence the way you feel by changing the way you think. There are several good books available if you are inclined to do self-support. CBT is a recognized therapy and many psychologists, counsellors and behavioural therapists provide a professional service (in many cases you are required to pay, although seek advice from your GP before doing so for advice and help on what type of help you may need). CBT works on the basis that people can teach themselves to change the way they think about their problems. As a therapy it has been known to help people with anger problems, anxiety, panic attacks, obsessive-compulsive behaviour, depression and strong emotions such as guilt and jealousy. CBT is an effective, drug-free way of dealing with everyday problems such as feelings of low self-esteem, relationship problems and feeling bad about yourself. Greenberger and Padesky (1995) have brought out a very popular book about CBT available from local libraries and bookshops that explains the therapy and its principles very well. There are also many British books, free leaflets and web-sites on CBT (see Resources, p. 135).

Practical ways of relieving stress and chilling out

Some of these chill-out ideas have been contributed by friends, nurses, doctors, massage therapists and people experienced in chilling. See which suggestions suit you.

A hot bath

A long soak in a hot bath with essential oils in the water (lavender and ylang ylang) can work wonders. Use candles to create atmosphere and burn essential oils if desired. Listen to music. When you get out, do some simple yoga exercises to help you relax, and play your favourite relaxing music.

The above can be supplemented with having a massage, eating chocolate, going to bed and doing other activities such as tai-chi.

Alexander technique

This is an easy way to adjust your posture and release tension without being in a special frame of mind or place. Sit upright in your chair. Consider your posture. How you are sitting? Are you tense anywhere? Try to focus on your tense areas and relax each place in turn by stretching the head upwards, keeping your feet firmly on the ground, your head upright and your limbs relaxed in an open posture that is designed to help you become relaxed, but keeping correct body posture (see Resources, p. 134).

Exercise

Taking exercise is a great stress-buster although the type of exercise depends on your ability, willingness and time! Exercise can take various forms, such as walking (up and down stairs works!). It can take place sitting in a chair or lying in a bed for example, the EXTEND programme for older infirm people. EXTEND is a registered charity which provides quality-assured training, accredited qualifications and best practice advice for teachers of recreational exercise to music for the over-sixties and those with special needs. For carers, exercise is an important part of life. Walking to the shops, from the car to the supermarket or just around the yard, garden or street will be beneficial. Exercise in groups such as Pilates, yoga or aerobic classes can also have a social component and be a useful way of meeting others. Exercise is good for our physical and mental health and a good discipline for making sure that we take care of ourselves and take time out to focus attention on our bodies.

The Expert Patients Programme

If you are living with or caring for someone with a long-term health condition, the Expert Patients Programme (EPP) can help provide you with essential tools to help you cope. The programme is currently only available in England, although this is likely to change in the future to expand into other parts of the UK. The programme is run by a not-for-profit organization and is designed to help carers and people with long-term illness to take more control of their lives. A typical programme runs over 6 weeks and is tailored to suit individual needs. Each weekly session is conducted by trained tutors, themselves carers or people living with long-term illness, many volunteer their services, and each session lasts approximately two to three hours. The topics covered within the sessions can include the following:

● managing pain and discomfort
● coping with tiredness and fatigue
● relaxation techniques, exercise and healthy eating
● improving communication between family and friends
● coping with depression.

You may be able to volunteer your services or wish to use the programme for help and support. For further details of the nearest local Expert Patients Programme, see the Resources section (p. 143).

Respite care

One of the most important kinds of support that friends and family can offer carers is respite care. This essential element of support is basically designed to give the carer a rest, a break and some respite from the hard and often emotionally draining task of providing full-time care. I recall that when my wife and I were caring for my father (who had cancer), we organized a variety of different sources of respite care, although we did not realize that it had a name. 'Respite care' is the term given to a vast range of supportive help and can take the form of coming round and spending time with the patient while the carer goes out or simply sits in another room and relaxes watching a favourite TV show. Respite in my case enabled my wife and I to go out to the cinema or for a drink on our own. In my case, respite care was loosely structured around what we needed. My brother would come round for two to three hours while we went out, or a friend of the family would take my father out to the pub, leaving my wife and I to relax (see Costello 1990 for more details). Respite can also extend to include the patient attending a day centre or luncheon club. In a more structured way carers can receive respite if the patient spends time in a hospice, nursing home or hospital, perhaps for a short one-week period. This type of care can be arranged by the social worker, community nurse or the carer and the family. Other organizations offering respite care are Crossroads care scheme (see Sources of help below and Resources, p. 140). Crossroads can arrange for a volunteer to visit your home and spend time with the patient, freeing the carer to do what they need to do for themselves: go swimming, attend an interview or go for a walk with a friend. Friends and family members can also arrange a short holiday break, over a weekend or longer, where the carer is able to take a more relaxed and substantive rest. Having a more long-term break can hep the care to 'recharge' their batteries and is a very positive way of helping the carer to become more effective in their caring role.

Friends and family are able to offer support in a variety of ways by looking for signs of tiredness in the carer, planning respite care before the carer becomes worn out, stressed and suffering from compassionate fatigue (see chapter 5). The following is a summary of the type of things family and friends can do to offer respite to the carer.

● Offer to take over and look after or spend time with the patient, freeing up the carer for a period of time.
● Take the patient out and leave the carer to do what they would like to do.
● Arrange a surprise day/night out to enable the carer to socialize and meet friends.
● Find out what interests or hobbies the carer has and arrange for them to go out to the theatre, cinema or attend a meeting.
● Organize a holiday break for the carer (this could involve the patient as well or be focused on a break just for the carer). Respite usually entails the carer having time to call their own!

● Ensure that the carer has regular time to call their own on a weekly basis. This way they can look forward to time when they can do the things they want to as well as having ad hoc time when they can take a much-needed break if life becomes difficult.

As the list above shows, respite care comes in many forms. Providing one-off respite is an excellent form of support, although anticipating a holiday and break is also very welcome. Respite support also gives the carer and patient a break from each other and this in itself has therapeutic value. Knowing it is available is also a clear sign that others are thinking of you, which is invaluable.

Sources of help

Self-help and support groups

Becoming part of a self-help support group may not appeal to everyone but it is a fantastic way of helping yourself and the person you care for. There are many different support groups in the UK. One of the best known is the Crossroads Caring for Carers organization (see Resources, p. 140). Crossroads have over 200 schemes across the country. They provide a wide range of services for carers, including care in the home (by paid, trained workers), that enables carers to take a break, have respite care and essentially take time out from their carer role. Crossroads provide advice and tangible support on a range of issues and is a very focused organization with a wealth of knowledge (many of the carers have personal and professional experience).

Another group to contact for information about local support groups in your area is the Patients' Association. You may find their helpline useful for putting you in touch with other local carer support groups. They also provide advice on how to make a complaint about local health services and provide advice on drawing up a living will (see Resources, p. 152).

Voluntary services

Many local authorities operate a range of voluntary services to help people get the best from their local, regional and national health services. One of the best ways to do this is through a national organization called the Council for Voluntary Services (CVS). CVS are able to offer advice and practical help on a range of locally available services, ranging from individual needs such as a need for a volunteer day/night sitter to referral to agencies offering specialist advice. CVS works by finding and putting you in touch with volunteers to help patients with disability and long-term problems live more independently. They do this by helping to develop volunteer programmes or organizing 'team tasks'. CVS works by recruiting people who wish to volunteer to do community work and aims to improve the lives of individuals by supporting them in the community. Much of their work relies on the generosity of companies, charitable trusts and individual supporters.

Patient Advice and Liaison Service (PALS)

PALS is an NHS service available from hospitals and health centres that can give on-the-spot help and advice about health care services. It is not a complaints service as such, although patients and carers can make their views known to the service if they are not satisfied with the care and treatment they have received. Primarily PALS is available to help patients to receive better services and sort out everyday health-related problems. This is achieved by listening to your concerns, helping to clarify the issues and exploring the various options available. PALS is an information-giving service covering health clinics, dentists, opticians, pharmacies and hospitals. PALS can also help people with long-term illness by helping them to become involved in the management of their own care. Access can be gained via the local hospital or through telephoning or emailing the service. It can also be accessed through the website or through Google (see Resources, p. 152).

Practical and financial support

Carers' grant

Many, although not all, local authorities have a carers' strategy (in addition to the national carers' strategy). This includes provision for providing carers with a small grant. The strategy outlines how the funds available to the local authority will be spent in relation to meeting the needs of local carers. You are advised to contact your local authority and ask to speak to the carers strategy officer. In some cases organizations offering support to carers can be provided with funds from the carers' grant (if they apply), to help set up specific services (usually of a practical nature) for carers. Each local authority is given a slice of the carers' grant. I would encourage carers to contact their local strategy officer and ask them how the carers' grant is being spent in their area.

Education

Half of all the 6 million carers in the UK, most of whom are female, are also in paid employment. At the same time, many carers juggle a range of domestic responsibilities. This can cause many challenges to your daily life, least of all developing and having a life of your own. You may find that as a carer there are no opportunities or time for you to take up education. Many carers enjoy education and learning, as well as the freedom this type of activity gives them to spend time with others. For further information on educational opportunities, contact your local social services department for funding for learning through the local authority's carers grants (also the Disability Rights Handbook, see Resources, p. 142). Social services departments may also be able to help you to find someone to take over your carer duties while you study.

The Carers (Equal Opportunities) Act 2004 came into force in April 2005 to ensure that carers are able to take up opportunities that people without caring responsibilities enjoy and take for granted. The Employment Act (2002) now gives working parents of disabled children under 18 the right to request flexible working arrangements. At the same time carers have the right to take unpaid time off for looking after dependants in emergency situations. Taking unpaid time off obviously affects you financially, but it is possible to receive payment for your role as a carer from the patient, who may be eligible for a range of benefits and allowances for people with long-term illnesses. Carers can also request an assessment of their needs under the 2004 act, which looks at their ability to continue in their caring role and what services the local authority can provide to support/sustain them in their role. Responsibility for carrying out this assessment lies with social services, who have the power to provide services – for example, carer breaks, respite care, further services for the disabled. These may be identified with the assessment. See your local authority website (under Health and Social Care) for further information.

Benefits for carers

The main benefit for carers is the Carers allowance. To qualify for this there are multiple rules, one of which is that the person you are caring for (child or adult) must be getting Attendance Allowance (at any rate), or the middle rate of Disability Living Allowance (see below). There are other tests. At the moment, there is an earnings threshold is £87.00 per week. One cannot be in full-time education, you must be caring for at least 35 hours a week and must be aged 16 or over. Details about these rules often change. They can be obtained from your local authority websites or through Social Services Department. For further information see the Carers Allowance Unit and Department of Health entries in the 'Resources and useful contacts' section.

Benefits available for people with long-term illness

There are a range of benefits available for people who have a long-term illness that also makes them disabled. These benefits are constantly being reviewed by the government and changes made alter the eligibility criteria and amount of benefit. The information pertaining to benefits was accurate up to going to press. However, things do change and it is always a good idea to seek expert up-to-date advice on your personal situation. Another useful source is the *Disability Rights Handbook*, which is currently in its 32nd edition. This is packed full of information advice on benefits and helpful suggestions on where to get sound professional advice on a range of issues affecting people with disabilities.

There are two main types of benefits for disabled people: Attendance Allowance (AA) and Disability Living Allowance (DLA). Both are non-means-tested and tax-free. Receiving either allowance should not reduce any other benefits. You cannot, however, claim both. Both benefits enable you to receive money to help with the costs of personal care. DLA also has a mobility component to help with getting around. If you are under 65 and need help with personal care, you can claim DLA.

Disability Living Allowance

To claim Disability Living Allowance (DLA), you must apply before your 65th birthday. There are no special rules for people who are already claiming DLA when they reach the age of 65. If you are aged 65 and over, need help with personal care (washing, dressing, toileting and bathing) and are claiming for the first time, you should claim Attendance Allowance (see below). There is also a backwards test for DLA, which means that you must have had needs for 3 months in the past and are likely to have them for 6 months in the future to qualify. DLA care is paid at three rates – Lower, Middle and Higher – and the mobility rate is paid at two, rates lower and higher. Some benefits may be increased if the patient is in receipt of Disability Living Allowance, Attendance Allowance and other means-tested awards such as income support and pension credit.

Attendance Allowance

If you have a long-term illness that makes you disabled and you require help with personal care, you should normally apply for Attendance Allowance (AA). There are two rates of AA – higher rate and lower rate – depending on the extent of help the patient requires. The amount you receive depends on how much help you need and the type of help. People with long-term illness are not automatically entitled to AA because they have a particular illness or disability. However, they can claim AA if they need help with personal care from another person or if they need someone to supervise or watch over them. They do not have to be actually getting help from anyone. What is important is that they need help and must have normally needed this help for 6 months. If it has not been for 6 months but they are likely to continue to need help for some time, claim immediately so that they can get AA as soon as you are entitled. If the person you care for has been diagnosed as being terminally ill, they can still apply for AA under special rules. They will automatically get the highest rate for the rest of their life without needing to fulfil any other conditions.

You can qualify for DLA as well as AA under special rules, for example, when death can reasonably be expected within a 6-month period. This means that the highest rate of AA or DLA is paid automatically after providing a DS1500 report for your GP or hospital consultant.

For further advice on benefits and allowances for people with a long-term illness, contact your local social services department or (if over 60) contact one of the charities such as Help the Aged (see Resources) for specific information. Useful advice can also be obtained from the many support groups, such as the Multiple Sclerosis Society (see Resources).

Summary

This chapter has attempted to convey the important message that carers are important and valued people who provide a service to others, but also need to be supported themselves. There are services such as the national Crossroads care schemes available to help and provide carers with support. These may be useful to some (but not all) carers. Some carers may wish to gain access and support from self-help groups. Groups of like-minded individuals who have a common purpose often find it reassuring to be amongst people who share similar experiences. Whatever form of support suits you as an individual, make sure that you avail yourself of this support on a regular basis. The quality of the support you receive can, and often does, influence the quality of care you provide for the patient. 'Caring for the carers' has long been a mantra amplified by some professionals who recognise the important role of the 6 million carers in the UK. However, turning the rhetoric into reality means providing resources and funding to ensure that current existing schemes can be maintained and expanded. At the same time it is important that new developments and initiatives receive recognition. Working in this way, as *Carers UK* do, may appeal to you, and if so may also provide the necessary encouragement you require to enable you to keep on caring. My final message to you as a carer is to look after yourself, physically and psychologically. Tell yourself when you look in the mirror in the morning that you do a great job, an important one, and that you are a valued and respected person – one in 6 million who are caring for someone else and making a commitment and a difference to someone else's life. On their behalf, thank you and keep on doing what you do.

References and further reading

Addington-Hall, J. & Higginson, I. (2001) *Palliative Care for non-cancer patients*. Oxford University Press, Oxford.

Barlow, W. (1975) *The Alexander Principle*. Arrow, London.

Becker, B. & Gamlin, R. (2006) *Fundamental Aspects of Palliative Care Nursing*. Banner Books, London.

Browne, M., Mahoney A. & Eochaidh, G.D. (2005) *Care of people dying in hospitals project*. Dublin, Eire: Irish Hospice Foundation.

Brykczynska, G. (1992) 'Caring – a dying art?' In *Nursing care: the challenge to change*, ed. M. Jolley & G. Brykczynska. Edward Arnold, London, pp. 1–45.

Buijssen, H. (2005) *The simplicity of Dementia: a guide for family and carers*. Jessica Kingsley, London.

Campling, F. & Sharpe, M. (2006) *Living with a long-term illness: the facts*. Oxford University Press, Oxford.

Cassidy, S. (1988) *Sharing the darkness: the spirituality of Caring*. Darton, Longman & Todd, London.

Chalder, T. (1999) *Coping with chronic fatigue*. Sheldon Press, London.

Copp, G. (1999) 'Facing impending death'. *Nursing Times Books*, London.

Costello, J. (1990) 'Dying at home'. *Nursing Times* 86(8), 49–52.

Costello, J. (1995) 'Helping relatives cope with the grieving process'. *Professional Nurse*, 11(2), 89–92.

Costello, J. (1996) 'Acknowledging loss: reflections on bereavement'. *Elderly Care* 8(4), 35–6.

Costello, J. (1997) 'The emotional cost of palliative care'. *European Journal of Palliative Care*, 3(4), 171–4.

Costello, J. (2004) 'Is it always ethical to tell the truth to cancer patients?'. *Cancer Nursing Practice* 8, 5–31.

Costello, J. (2004) *Nursing the dying patient: caring in different contexts.* Palgrave, London.

Costello, J. (2006) 'Dying well: nurses' experiences of good and bad deaths in hospital'. *Journal of Advanced Nursing* 54(5), 1–8.

Costello, J. & Hargreaves, S. (1998) 'Anticipatory grief: some implications for social work practice in working with families facing impending loss'. *Practice* 10(3), 45–54.

Department of Health (2000) *The NHS Cancer Plan: a plan for investment, a plan for reform.* Department of Health, London.

Department of Health (2001) *Treatment choice in psychological therapies and counselling.* Department of Health, London.

Department of Health (2004) *Preferred place of care.* Department of Health, London.

Ellershaw, J. & Ward, C. (2003) 'Care of the dying patient: the last hours or days of life'. *British Medical Journal* 326, 30–4.

Fallowfield, L. & Jenkins, V. (1999) 'Effective communication skills are the key to good cancer care'. *European Journal of Cancer* 35, 1592–7.

Fontana, D. (2004) *Meditation week by week.* Duncan Baird Publishers, London.

Greaves, I. (2007) *Disability Rights Handbook* (32nd edition). Disability Alliance, London.

Greenberger, D. & Padeslky, C.A. (1995) *Mind over mood.* The Guilford Press, New York.

Griffin, A.P. (1981) 'A philosophical analysis of caring in nursing'. *Journal of Advanced Nursing* 8(4), 289–95.

Highfield, M.E. (2004) 'Providing spiritual care to patients with cancer'. *Clinical Journal of Oncology Nursing* 4(3), 115–20.

Holman, H. & Lorig, K. (2000) 'Patients as partners in managing chronic disease'. *British Medical Journal* 320, 526–7.

Horn, S. & Munafo, M. (1997) *Pain: theory research and Intervention.* Open University Press, Buckingham.

Illich, I. (2002) *Limits to medicine medical nemesis: the expropriation of health.* Marion Boyars Publishers, London.

Kubler-Ross, E. (1991) *On death and dying.* Double Day, New York.

Lloyd-Williams, M. (2004) 'Emotions and cognitions: psychological aspects of care'. In *Palliative Care Nursing*, ed. S. Payne, J. Seymour & C. Ingleton. Open University Press, Oxford. pp. 299–311.

Mackereth, P. & Carter, A. (2006) *Massage and Bodywork: adapting therapies for cancer.* Churchill Livingstone, Elsevier, London.

McNamara, B., Waddell, C. & Colvin, M. (1995) 'Threats to the good death: the cultural context of stress and coping among hospice nurses'. *Sociology of Health and Illness* 17(2), 222–44.

Mowrey, B.D. (1993) *Herbal tonic therapies*. Keats Publishing, Hartford, Connecticut.

Newton, E. (1980) *This bed my center*. Virago, London.

NICE (2004) Anxiety: management of anxiety (panic disorder, with or without agoraphobia, and generalised anxiety disorder) in adults in primary, secondary and community care. http://www.nice.org.uk/Guidance/CG22 (accessed 4 February 2009).

NICE (2004) Depression: management of depression in primary and secondary care. NICE Guideline December 2004. http://www.nice.org.uk/CG023 (accessed 4 February 2009).

Oliver, D. (2006) *Motor Neurone Disease: a family affair*. Sheldon Press, London.

Ostrom, N. (1993) *America's biggest cover-up: 50 more things everyone should know about the Chronic Fatigue Syndrome epidemic and its link to AIDS*. That New Magazine.

Parkes, C.M. (1972) *Bereavement: studies of grief in adult life*. Penguin, Harmondsworth.

Payne, S., Horn, S. & Relf, M. (1999) *Loss and bereavement*. Open University Press, Buckingham.

Roach, S.M. (1985) 'A foundation for nursing ethics'. In *Nursing law and ethics*, ed. I. Carmi & S. Scheider. Berlin, Springer Verlag, pp. 170–1.

Rogers, A., Karlsen, S. & Addington-Hall, J. (2000) 'All the services were excellent. It is when the human element comes in that things go wrong: dissatisfaction with hospital care at the end of life'. *Journal of Advanced Nursing* 31(4), 768–74.

Ronning, R. (2003) 'The importance of care as a positive concept'. *Quality in Ageing* 3(4), 34–43.

Rose, D.B. (1988) *Essential Psychiatry*. Blackwell Scientific, London.

Saunders, C. (1970) 'The nature and management of terminal pain'. In *Matters of life and death*, ed. Camps *et al*. Darton, Longman & Todd, London, pp. 15–26.

Seale, C. (1991) 'Communication and awareness about death: a study of a random sample of dying people'. *Social Science and Medicine* 32, 943–52.

Seale, C. & Kelly, M. (1997) 'A comparison of hospital and hospice care for people who die: news of supporting spouse'. *Palliative Medicine* 11, 93–100.

Skilbeck, J. & Payne, S. (2003) 'Emotional support and the role of clinical nurse specialists in palliative care'. *Journal of Advanced Nursing* 43(5), 521–530.

Smith, R. (2000) 'Good death. Editorial'. *British Medical Journal* 7228 (15 January), 129.

Sontag, S. (2001) *Illness as metaphor and AIDS as a metaphor.* Picador, New York.

Taylor, B. (1993) 'Hospice nurses tell their stories about a good death: the value of storytelling as a qualitative health research method'. *Annual Review of Health Social Science*, 3, 97–108.

Trickett, S. (2001) *Coping with anxiety and depression.* Sheldon Press, London.

Twycross, R. (2003) *Introducing palliative care.* Radcliffe Medical Press, Oxford.

Vachon, L.M.S. (1999) 'Dying patients are not the real problem'. In *Occupational stress in the care of the critically ill, the dying and the bereaved*, ed. L.M.S. Vachon. Hemisphere, Washington DC, 51–74.

Walter, J.A. (1994) *The revival of death.* Routledge, London.

Watson, M., Lucas, C., Hoy, A. & Back, I. (2005) *Oxford handbook of palliative care.* Oxford University Press, Oxford.

Williams, C.J. (2001) Overcoming Depression: A Five Areas Approach. Hodder Arnold, London. http://apt.rcpsych.org/cgi/content/full/8/3/172 (accessed 4 February 2009).

World Health Organization (1996) *Cancer pain relief*, 2nd edition, WHO, Geneva.

Yardley, L., Donovan-Hall, M., Francis, K. & Todd, C. (2006) 'Older people's views of advice about falls prevention: a qualitative study', *Health Education Research* 21(4), 508–17.

The 'Overcoming' Series, Constable and Robinson, London.

A large series of self-help books that use the theories and concepts of CBT to help people overcome many common problems. Titles include: *Overcoming social anxiety and shyness, Overcoming depression* and *Overcoming low self-esteem.*

Resources and useful contacts

Advisory Center for Education (ACE)

A national charity that provides independent advice for parents and carers of children aged 5-16 in state-funded education. ACE aims to provide the information, support and high-quality advice that parents need to help their children at school, particularly where there are problems. ACE offers free advice on many subjects like exclusion from school, bullying, special educational needs and school admission appeals.

Advisory Centre for Education (ACE)
1c Aberdeen Studios
22 Highbury Grove
London N5 2DQ
Tel: 0808 800 5793
Email: enquiries@ace-ed.org.uk
Website: www.ace-ed.org.uk

Alexander Principle (The) (stress relief)

The Society of Teachers of the Alexander Technique – STAT – was established in 1958 and is the internationally recognized representative body. The Society has over 1500 members world-wide with more than 850 teaching members in the UK. They are professionally qualified and adhere to a published code of ethics.

The Society of Teachers of the Alexander Technique
1st Floor, Linton House
39-51 Highgate Road
London NW5 1RS

Tel: 0845 230 7828
Email: office@stat.org.uk
Website: www.stat.org.uk

Alzheimer's Society

Advice on many physical, social and emotional aspects of the disease and benefits available
Alzheimer's Society.
Devon House
58 St Katharine's Way
London E1W 1JX
Tel: 020 7423 3500
Helpline: 0845 300 0336
Email: enquiries@alzheimers.org.uk
Website: www.alzheimers.org.uk
Scotland helpline: 0808 808 3000
Scotland website: www.alzscot.org

Beating the Blues

Beating the Blues is a computerized cognitive behavioural therapy (CCBT) programme for depression and anxiety. It has been shown to be a cost effective and time efficient way of helping people suffering from these conditions to get better and stay better.
Ultrasis UK LTD
2nd Floor Northburgh House
10 Northburgh Street
London EC1V 0AT
Tel: 020 7566 3900
Email: ultrasis@ultrasis.com
Website: www.ultrasis.com

Breakthrough Breast Cancer

Breakthrough Breast Cancer is a charity registered in England, Wales and Scotland that provides people with free information help and advice about breast cancer and its prevention.
Breakthrough Breast Cancer
246 High Holborn
London WC1V 7EX
Tel: 020 7025 2400

Email: info@breakthrough.org.uk
Website: www.breakthrough.org.uk

The Bristol Approach

A leading UK charity specializing in the Bristol Approach to cancer care for people with cancer and those close to them. The Bristol Approach works hand-in-hand with medical treatment, offering a unique combination of physical, emotional and spiritual support, using complementary therapies and self-help techniques.
Penny Brohn Cancer Care (formerly *Bristol Cancer Help Centre*)
Penny Brohn Cancer Care
Chapel Pill Lane
Pill
Bristol BS20 0HH
Helpline: 0845 123 2310
Tel: 01275 370 100
Email: helpline@pennybrohn.org
Email: info@pennybrohn.org
Website: www.pennybrohncancercare.org

British Association for Behavioural and Cognitive Psychotherapies (BABCP)

The BABCP is the lead organization for Cognitive Behavioural Therapy in the UK.
BABCP
Victoria Buildings
9-13 Silver Street
Bury BL9 0EU
Tel: 0161 797 4484
Email: babcp@babcp.com
Website: www.babcp.com

British Association for Counselling and Psychotherapy

This is a service designed to enable potential clients to find a suitable counsellor with whom they feel comfortable, in their particular area.
BACP House
15 St John's Business Park
Lutterworth LE17 4HB

Tel: 01455 883300
Email: enquiries@bacp.co.uk
Website: www.bacp.co.uk

Cancerbackup

Cancerbackup has merged with **Macmillan Cancer Support,** to provide a wealth of high-quality, expertly developed information about cancer.
3 Bath Place
Rivington Street
London EC2A 3JR
Helpline: 0808 8001234
Website: www.cancerbackup.org.uk

Cancerlink

Provide information resource services to cancer patients, family and carers about a huge range of different types of cancer.
17 Britannia Street
London WC1X 9JN
Tel: 0171 833 2451
Website: http://www.njh.u-net.com/cancer.html

Carer's Allowance Unit

Carer's Allowance is a government benefit which can be claimed by carers who are 16 or over and care for a disabled person for at least 35 hours per week. The disabled person has to be in receipt of a qualifying benefit and the carer's earnings are taken into account. Contact the number below for details or to receive an information booklet and claim pack, or claim online on the website.
Carer's Allowance Unit
Palatine House
Lancaster Road
Preston PR1 1HB
Helpline: 01253 856 123
Website: www.direct.gov.uk

Carers UK

Campaigning group for better services and support for carers. Also involved in training carers.

Carers UK
20 Great Dover Street
London SE1 4LX
Helpline: 0808 808 7777
Tel: 020 7378 4999
Email: info@carersuk.org
Website: www.carersuk.org

Carers Scotland
91 Mitchell Street
Glasgow G1 3LN
Tel: 0141 221 9141
Email: info@carerscotland.org
Website: www.carerscotland.org

Carers Wales
River House
Ynysbridge Court
Gwaelod-y-Garth
Cardiff CF15 9SS
Tel: 029 2081 1370
Email: info@carerswales.org
Website: www.carerswales.org

Carers Northern Ireland
58 Howard Street
Belfast BT1 6PJ
Tel: 028 9043 9843
Email: info@carersni.org
Website: www.carersni.org

Cognitive Behavioural Therapy

For further information on Cognitive Behavioural Therapy visit the
following website:
Website: www.psychnet-uk.com/psychotherapy/psychotherapy_
cognitive_behavioural_therapy.htm.

Colostomy Association

Information, advice and support about a wide range of colostomies.
Colostomy Association

Head Office
2 London Court
East Street
Reading RG1 4QL
Tel: 0118 939 1537
Helpline: 0800 587 6744 *or* 0800 328 4257
Email: cass@colostomyassociation.org.uk
Website: www.colostomyassociation.org.uk

Compassionate Friends

The Compassionate Friends (TCF) is an organization of bereaved
parents and their families offering understanding, support and
encouragement to others after the death of a child or children. They
also offer support, advice and information to other relatives, friends
and professionals who are helping the family.
The Compassionate Friends (TCF)
53 North Street
Bristol BS3 1EN
Helpline: 0845 123 2304
Tel: 0845 120 3785
Helpline email: helpline@tcf.org.uk
Email: info@tcf.org.uk
Website: www.tcf.org.uk

Counsel and Care

Counsel and Care is a national charity working with older people,
their families and carers to get the best care and support. They provide
personalized, in-depth advice and information, which informs their
research and campaigning work.
Counsel and Care
Twyman House
16 Bonny Street
London NW1 9PG
Advice line: 0845 300 7585
Tel: 020 7241 8555
Email: advice@counselandcare.org.uk
Website: www.counselandcare.org.uk/

Crossroads Care Scheme

Crossroads' service is about giving time – improving the lives of carers by giving them a break from their caring responsibilities. They provide a reliable, tailored service for each carer and the person they care for with schemes in most parts of England and Wales. (See below for the websites for Crossroads' sister operations in Scotland and Northern Ireland.)

Crossroads Care Scheme
10 Regent Place
Rugby CV21 2PN
Tel: 0845 450 0350
Website: www.crossroads.org.uk/
Scotland website: www.crossroads-scotland.co.uk
Northern Ireland website: www.crossroadscare.co.uk

Cruse: Bereavement Care

Cruse Bereavement Care exists to promote the well-being of bereaved people and to enable anyone bereaved by death to understand their grief and cope with their loss. Services are free to bereaved people. The charity provides support and offers information, advice, education and training services.

Cruse Bereavement Care
PO Box 800
Richmond
Surrey TW9 1RG
Tel: 020 8939 9530
Helpline: 0844 477 9400
Young Person's freephone helpline: 0808 808 1677
Helpline email: helpline@cruse.org.uk
Email: info@cruse.org.uk
Website: www.crusebereavementcare.org.uk

Northern Ireland Regional Office
Piney Ridge, Knockbracken Healthcare Park
Saintfield Road
Belfast BT8 8BH.
Tel: 028 90 792419
Email: northern.ireland@cruse.org.uk

Cruse Bereavement Care Cymru
Ty Energlyn, Heol Las
Caerphilly/ Caerffili
CF83 2TT
Tel: 029 2088 6913
Email: wales.cymru@cruse.org.uk

Cruse Bereavement Care Scotland
Riverview House
Friarton Road
Perth PH2 8DF
Tel: 01738 444 178
Email: info@crusescotland.org.uk
Website: www.crusescotland.org.uk

Department for Work and Pensions

Promotes opportunity and independence for all; helps individuals achieve their potential through employment; works to end poverty in all its forms.
Website: www.dwp.gov.uk

Benefit enquiry line (disability benefits)
Tel: 0800 882200 (0800 220674 in Northern Ireland)
Textphone: 0800 24 3 3 55 (0800 24 37 87 in N Ireland)

Carers Allowance Unit
Tel: 01772 899729 (028 9090 6186 in Northern Ireland)

Working tax credit helpline
Tel: 0845 300 3900 (0845 603 2000 in Northern Ireland)
Textphone: 0845 300 3909 (0845 607 6078 in Northern Ireland)
If you need a form or help in Welsh, call 0845 302 1489.

Department of Health

Providing advice, support, guidance and publications on health and social policy.
Website: www.dh.gov.uk/en/index.htm

In particular, it is useful to look at the following reports/publications:
Saving Lives: Our Healthier Nation (1998)
Making a Difference (1999)
Various National Service Frameworks, in particular:

National Service Framework for Long-Term Conditions (2005)
The Expert Patient (2001)
Liberating the Talents (2002)
Chronic Disease Management Compendium (2004)
Improving Chronic Disease Management (2004)
NHS and Social Care Model (2005)
Caring for People with Long-term Conditions (2006)
Our Health, Our Care, Our Say (2006)
Supporting People with Long-term Conditions (2006)

Dial UK

DIAL UK is a national organization for a network of approximately 120 local Disability Information and Advice Line services (DIALs) run by and for disabled people.
DIAL UK
St Catherine's Tickhill Road
Doncaster DN4 8QN
Tel (voice and text): 01302 310123
Email: informationenquiries@dialuk.org.uk
Website: www.dialuk.info

Disability Alliance

Provides information for people with disabilities, covering a range of issues including social security benefits and tax credits. The Alliance also runs a dedicated telephone helpline for members only. (The Alliance currently has over 400 member organizations that are both local and national in their scope.) The Alliance plays an important role in advising and lobbying MPs on the effects of new and existing disability benefits.
Disability Alliance
Universal House
88–94 Wentworth Street
London E1 7SA
Tel (voice and text): 0207 247 8776
Email: office.da@dial.pipex.com
Website: www.disabilityalliance.org

Disability Rights Commission

The Disability Rights Commission has one key goal: "A society where all disabled people can participate fully as equal citizens". Since September 2007 it has merged with the Equality and Human Rights Commission. For help and advice contact their helplines:

0845 604 6610 (England)

0845 604 5510 (Scotland)

0845 604 8810 (Wales)

Website: www.equalityhumanrights.com

Disabled Living Foundation

A national charity that provides free, impartial advice about all types of daily living equipment and mobility products for disabled adults and children, older people, their carers and families.

Disabled Living Foundation

380-384 Harrow Road

London W9 2HU

Helpline: 0845 130 9177 (textphone 020 7432 8009)

Tel: 0171 289 6111

Email: advice@dlf.org.uk or info@dlf.org.uk

Website: www.dlf.org.uk

Employers for Carers

Set up with support from Carers UK, it is a membership forum for employers who want to support the people in their workforce who are carers. Its purpose is: to identify and promote the business benefits of supporting carers in the workplace; influence employment policy and practice to create a culture which supports carers in and into work; provide a service to employers seeking to develop best practice in the workplace. It has been set up with support from Carers UK.

Tel: 0207 378 4940

Email: Mark.Murphy@carersuk.org

Website: www.carersuk.org/Employersforcarers

Expert Patients Programme (EPP)

The Expert Patients Programme is a lay-led self-management programme specifically developed for people living with long-term conditions.

Tel: 01886 833186 (Sharon Wong at EPP)

Website: www.dh.gov.uk/en/Aboutus/
MinistersandDepartmentLeaders/ChiefMedicalOfficer/
ProgressOnPolicy/ProgressBrowsableDocument /DH_4102757

Family Fund

The Family Fund helps families with severely disabled children to have choices and the opportunity to enjoy ordinary life. They give grants for things that make life easier and more enjoyable for the disabled child and their family, such as washing machines, driving lessons, hospital visiting costs, computers and holidays.
Family Fund
Unit 4, Alpha Court
Monks Cross Drive
Huntington, York YO32 9WN
Tel: 0845 130 4542 or 01904 621115
Email: info@familyfund.org.uk
Website: www.familyfund.org.uk

FearFighter

FearFighter is a new method for delivering CBT (Cognitive Behavioural Therapy) via a computer (standalone PC or internet). Approved by The National Institute of Clinical Excellence (NICE) and included by the NHS in the guidance for the treatment of Anxiety and Phobia, FearFighter is accessed by referral from your GP, Health Worker or in some cases directly via self referral.
CCBT Ltd
Tudor Court
14 Edward Street
Birmingham B1 2RX
TEL: 0121 233 2873
Email: enquiries@fearfighter.com
Website: www.fearfighter.com

(Please note: free access can only be prescribed by your doctor in England and Wales.)

Help the Aged

Useful information on a wide range of topics including financial, tax, bereavement, healthy eating, security, care homes and thinking about money. (See 'SeniorLine' entry)

Website: www.helptheaged.org.uk
Help the Aged – England
207–221 Pentonville Road
London N1 9UZ
Tel: 0207 278 1116
Email: info@helptheaged.org.uk

Help the Aged – Scotland
11 Granton Square
Edinburgh EH5 1HX
Tel: 0131 551 6331
Email: infoscot@helptheaged.org.uk

Help the Aged – Wales
12 Cathedral Rd
Cardiff CF11 9LJ
Tel: 02920 346 550
Email: infocymru@helptheaged.org.uk

Help the Aged – Northern Ireland
Ascot House
Shaftesbury Square
Belfast BT2 7DB
Tel: 02890 230 666
Email: infoni@helptheaged.org.uk

Help the Hospices

Leading charity supporting hospice care throughout the UK. The
web site is full of information, support and advice for patients and
professional staff.
Hospice House
34–44 Britannia Street
London WC1X 9JG
Tel: 020 7520 8200
Email: info@helpthehospices.org.uk
Website: www.helpthehospices.org.uk

Hospice Information Service (HIS)

The HIS publishes a directory of hospice and palliative care services
and is provided in partnership with St Christopher's Hospice. Send a
large SAE with three first-class stamps for written information.

St Christopher's Hospice
51 Lawrie Park Road
Sydenham
London SE26 6DL
Tel: 020 778 9252 or 020 7520 8222 (at Help the Hospices)
Email: info@hospiceinformation.info
Website: www.stchristophers.org.uk
Website: www.hospiceinformation.info

Individual Complaint Advocacy Service (ICAS)

This service supports patients and their carers wishing to pursue a complaint about their NHS treatment or care. It was launched in 2003 and provides for the first time a national service delivered to agreed quality standards. See website for local contacts:
http://www.dh.gov.uk/en/Policyandguidance/Organisationpolicy/
Complaintspolicy/NHScomplaintsprocedure/DH_4087428

KOSH.COM

Conversations to Remember is a DVD of people with life limiting illness and how they cope. It is an intimate portrayal of how people with life-threatening conditions and carers carry on with their lives, giving a voice to those people who are rarely heard.
The Kosh
59 Stapleton Hall Road
London N4 3QF
Tel: 020 8374 0407
Email: info@thekosh.com
Website: www.thekosh.com

Lawpack (for living wills)

Lawpack, the UK's DIY legal publisher, offers a range of do-it-yourself legal guides, legal kits and legal forms to help you resolve your legal issues and save legal fees.
Lawpack
76-89 Alscot Road
London SE1 3AW
Tel: 020 7394 4040
Website: www.lawpack.co.uk

Learn Direct

Learn Direct offers flexible courses so that you can do many courses at your local centre or from home or work if you have access to the Internet. Courses are broken down into bite-sized chunks, so people can learn at their own pace whenever and wherever it suits them.
Learn Direct
PO Box 900
Leicester LE1 6ER
Tel: 0800 100900 or 0800 101 901
Website: www.learndirect.co.uk

Living Life to the Full

Free online life skills course for people feeling distressed and their carers. Helps people understand how they feel and helps them make changes in their thinking, activities, sleep and relationships.
Website: www.livinglifetothefull.com

Macmillan Nurses (and Macmillan Cancer Support)

Macmillan exists to help improve the lives of people living with cancer and their families and carers. One in three people get cancer and we are all affected in some way.
Macmillan Cancer Support
89 Albert Embankment
London SE1 7UQ
Helpline: 0808 8082020
Youth Helpline (aged 12-21): 0808 808 0800
Tel: 020 7840 7840
Website: www.macmillan.org.uk

Marie Curie Cancer Care

Marie Curie Nurses provide free nursing care to patients with cancer as well as those with other non-cancer conditions in their own homes.
Website: www.mariecurie.org.uk
Marie Curie Cancer Care – England
89 Albert Embankment
London SE1 7TP
Tel: 020 7599 7777

Marie Curie Cancer Care – Scotland
14 Links Place
Edinburgh EH6 7EB
Tel: 0131 561 3900

Marie Curie Cancer Care – Wales
Block C Mamhilad House
Mamhilad Park Estate
Pontypool
Torfaen NP4 0HZ
Tel: 01495 740827

Marie Curie Cancer Care – Northern Ireland
60 Knock Road
Belfast BT5 6LQ
Tel: 028 9088 2060

MedicAlert

A registered charity providing a life-saving identification system to
protect and save lives. It can communicate your Living Will directly
to doctors in an emergency.
MedicAlert
1 Bridge Wharf
156 Caledonian Road
London N1 9UU
Tel: 0800 581420 or 020 7833 3034
Email: info@medicalert.org.uk
Website: www.medicalert.org.uk

Mood Gym

Information, quizzes, games and skills training to help prevent
depression.
Website: www.moodgym.anu.edu.au

Motor Neurone Disease Association

The Motor Neurone Disease (MND) Association is the only national
organization in England, Wales and Northern Ireland dedicated to
the support of people with MND and those who care for them. *MND
Connect* offers advice, practical and emotional support and directing
to other services and agencies. The service is for people living with
MND, carers, family members, Health and Social Care Professionals

and Association staff and volunteers who directly support people
with MND
Motor Neurone Disease Association
PO Box 246
Northampton NN1 2PR
MND Connect tel: 08457 626262
Tel: 01604 250505
Email: enquiries@mndassociation.org
Email MND Connect: mndconnect@mndassociation.org
Website: www.mndassociation.org

Multiple Sclerosis Society

The MS society has a carers' opportunity fund available for carers of
people with MS. The fund is available for carers who wish to pursue
educational opportunities and receive financial support. Contact the
grants team on 0250 84380700, or see the website for an application
form.
Email: helpline@mssociety.org.uk
Website: www.mssociety.org.uk

MS National Centre – England
372 Edgware Road
London NW2 6ND
Tel: 0808 800 8000

MS National Centre – Scotland
Ratho Park
88 Glasgow Road, Ratho Station
Newbridge EH28 8PP
Tel: 0131 335 4050

Multiple Sclerosis Society Wales/Cymru
Temple Court
Cathedral Road
Cardiff CF11 9HA
Tel: 029 2078 6676

Multiple Sclerosis Society – Northern Ireland
The Resource Centre
34 Annadale Avenue
Belfast BT7 3JJ
Tel: 02890 802 802

National Institute for Health and Clinical Excellence (NICE)

Independent health organization providing guidance on best treatment and practice.
NICE
MidCity Place
71 High Holburn
London WC1V 6NA
Tel: 0207 067 5800
Email: nice@nice.org.uk
Website: www.nice.org.uk

(Manchester Office)
National Institute for Health and Clinical Excellence
Level 1A, City Tower
Piccadilly Plaza
Manchester M1 4BD
Tel: 0845 003 7780

NHS Direct

The NHS information service covers a wide range of issues on its freephone information lines:
Helpline: 0845 46 47
Website: www.nhsdirect.nhs.uk
For Scotland only:
Helpline: 08454 24 24 24
Website: www.nhs24.com

Open University

Available to get a qualification that will help you develop, change your career, or learn a subject in depth. For most courses you don't need any previous qualifications. The OU have a world-leading blend of supported open learning and innovative course materials.
The Open University
PO Box 197
Milton Keynes MK7 6BJ
Tel: 01908 653231 or 01908 274066
Enquiry helpline: 0845 300 60 90
Website: www.open.ac.uk

Parkinson's Disease Society

The national leading charity for information about services, research and carer information on Parkinson's disease.
PDS National Office
215 Vauxhall Bridge Road
London SW1V 1ET
Tel: 0207 931 8080
Helpline: 0808 800 0303
Email: enquiries@parkinsons.org.uk
Website: www.parkinsons.org.uk

The Parkinson's Disease Society Scottish Office
Forsyth House
Lomond Court
Castle Business Park
Stirling FK9 4TU
Tel: 01786 433811
Email: pds.scotland@parkinsons.org.uk

The Parkinson's Disease Society Welsh Office
Maritime Offices
Woodland Terrace
Maesycoed
Pontypridd CF37 1DZ
Tel: 01443 404916
Email: pds.wales@parkinsons.org.uk

The Parkinson's Disease Society Northern Ireland Office
14 Linen Mill Grove
Edenderry
Belfast BT8 8GX
Tel: 0844 225 3680
Email: nmoore@parkinsons.org.uk
YPN (Younger Parkinson's Network)
PO Box 33209
London SW1V 1WH
Tel: 0808 800 0303
Website: http://yap-web.net/

Patient Advice and Liaison Service (PALS)

Contact PALS online or phone your local hospital, clinic, GP surgery or health centre and ask for details of the PALS, or try NHS Direct on 0845 46 47.
www.dh.gov.uk/en/Policyandguidance/Organisationpolicy/
PatientAndPublicinvolvement/Patientadviceandliaisonservices/
index.htm

Patients Association

An excellent source of help, with news, updates, chatroom and a wealth of information about and for carers. The trust is the largest provider of comprehensive carers' support services in the UK with 129 independently managed Carers' Centres and interactive websites: Carers.org and YC Net. The Trust currently provides quality information advice and support services to 290,000 carers, including just over 15,000 young carers.
The Patients Association
PO BOX 935
Harrow HA1 3YJ
Helpline: 08456 08 4455
Email: helpline@patients-association.com
Website: www.patients-association.com

Relate

Help, confidential advice and support on relationship matters.
Tel: 0300 100 1234
Website: www.relate.org.uk

The Royal British Legion

The legion provides financial social and emotional support to millions who have or who are currently serving in the armed forces and their dependents. Currently nearly 10.5 million people are eligible for our support.
The Royal British Legion
199 Borough High Street
London SE1 1AA
Tel: 020 3207 2100 or 08457 725 725
Website: www.britishlegion.org.uk (for Scotland: www.rblscotland.org.uk)

The Royal National Institute of Blind People (RNIB)

National UK charity providing a good range of information for blind or partially sighted people. RNIB offer advice and help to people with sight difficulties on disability benefits. See also your local social services departments who have teams of specialist who offer help.

Royal National Institute of Blind People
105 Judd Street
London WC1H 9NE
Helpline: 0845 766 9999
Tel: 020 7388 1266
Email: helpline@rnib.org.uk
Website: www.rnib.org.uk

The Royal National Institute for Deaf People (RNID)

RNID offers advice and help to people with hearing difficulties on disability benefits. See also your local social services department who have teams of specialist who offer help.

RNID
19–23 Featherstone Street
London ECIY 8SL
Helpline: 0808 808 0123
Tel: 020 7296 8000
Website: www.rnid.org.uk

RNID Scotland
Empire House
131 West Nile Street
Glasgow G1 2RX
Tel: 0141 341 5330
Email: rnidscotland@rnid.org.uk

RNID Wales
16 Cathedral Road
Cardiff CF11 9LJ
Tel: 029 2033 3034
Email: rnidcymru@rnid.org.uk

RNID Northern Ireland
Wilton House
5 College Square North
Belfast BT1 6AR

Telephone or textphone: 028 9023 9619
Text answerphone: 028 9031 2033
Email: information.nireland@rnid.org.uk

Samaritans

Samaritans provides confidential, non-judgmental, emotional support 24 hours a day for people who are experiencing feelings of distress or despair, including those which could lead to suicide. Samaritans is available to anyone in the UK and Ireland. If you live outside of the UK and Ireland, visit www.befrienders.org to find your nearest helpline. Write to us at:
Chris
PO Box 9090
Stirling FK8 2SA
Helpline: 08457 90 90 90
Republic of Ireland Helpline: 1850 60 90 90
Email: Jo@samaritans.org
Website: www.samaritans.org

SeniorLine

SeniorLine is a free welfare rights advice service for older people and their carers run by Help the Aged. Trained advice workers can offer advice or information about a wide range of issues including community/residential care, welfare/disability benefits and housing.
Tel: 0808 8006565
Textphone: 0800 269626 (0808 808 7575 in Northern Ireland)
Email: seniorline@helptheaged.org.uk
Website: www.helptheaged.org.uk/advice/advice.html

Terrence Higgins Trust

For AIDS patients, people who are HIV positive and their families.
Terrence Higgins Trust
52–54 Grays Inn Road
London WC1X 8JU
Helpline: 0845 12 21 200
Tel: 020 832 0330
Email: info@tht.org.uk
Website: www.tht.org.uk

University of the Third Age (U3A)

The Third Age Trust is the national representative body for the Universities of Third Age (U3As) in the UK. U3As are self-help, self-managed lifelong learning co-operatives for older people no longer in full time work, providing opportunities for their members to share learning experiences in a wide range of interest groups and to pursue learning not for qualifications, but for fun.

The Third Age Trust
Old Municipal Buildings
19 East Street
Bromley BR1 1QE
Tel: 0208 466 6139 or 020 8315 0199
Website: www.u3a.org.uk

Glossary

advanced decision (also known as Living Will) document: legally enforceable document usually written at or towards the end of life, which relates to the patient's wishes when their condition becomes terminal.

Agnostic: a person who believes that we know nothing of things beyond those which we are able to see.

ascites: accumulation of fluid in the abdominal cavity caused by a number of problems related to liver damage to tumours of the pancreas and gall bladder.

asthma: a respiratory problem caused by both allergic reactions to various proteins (such as grass, pollen, animal hair) or brought on by internal factors (like stress and anxiety). Acute attacks can occur at any time and the condition can last for many years and become long-term.

atheists: someone who does not believe in the existence of a god.

atherosclerosis: generally used to mean 'hardening of the arteries'. More common in older people, although not exclusive, as it can occur in younger people due to changes on the inside of the artery narrowing the artery and leading to circulatory problems often high blood pressure (hypertension).

Chronic Fatigue Syndrome (CFS): a long-term illness or syndrome characterized by constant, overwhelming fatigue, lymphadenopathy (inflammation of the lymph glands), headache, myalgia, arthralgia, memory loss.

Chronic Obstructive Airways Disease (COPD): A long-term degenerative disease of the respiratory system, called *Chronic Bronchitis* in the past, that may include **emphysema** and **asthma**. Associated with smoking and made worse by smoking and living in polluted environments. The person has difficulty breathing on exertion, such as when getting out of bed, washing and walking. It is very anxiety-provoking and patients require oxygen to relieve their breathing difficulties.

cyanosis: the blue appearance seen in people with breathing problems. Often the extremities are cold and appear blue – ears, lips, hands, toes, fingers – due to poor circulation of oxygen around the body.

decubitus ulcer: another term for pressure sore, which is skin breakdown caused by pressure in areas of bony prominence in the body.

emotional IQ: the ability within one person to engage with others sufficiently to perceive their emotional state (and sometimes the reason for that emotional state) and emotional needs, and to use that understanding to drive their thinking, their behaviour and their management of the relationship.

emphysema: an abnormality of lung tissue where air or gas is found in the lung tissue. Can be caused by surgery or due to recurring respiratory problems making it difficult for the person to breathe properly with symptoms similar to COPD.

holistic: care that takes into account the person's physical, psychological, social and spiritual well-being; extended to include the person's relatives.

humidifier: machine used for delivering drugs used in people with breathing problems (via a small motor), providing relief from episodes of breathlessness. Should not be used regularly without medical advice. Can be borrowed from health centres or Red Cross organizations. Can also be purchased – ask your chemist.

Multi-Infarct Dementia: (MID) is well-known. In this case, small brain infarcts cause oxygen loss to parts of the brain, causing tissue erosion.

NSAIDs: non-steroidal anti-inflammatory drugs.

Opioid drugs: drugs used to control pain that are morphine-based, including morphine.

palliative (palliative care): treatment and care given when there is no realistic hope of a cure but the quality of a person's life can be improved by providing effective interventions.

Parenteral Feeding line or Total Parenetral Nutrition (TPN): device is similar to an intravenous line which is inserted into the vein. Sometimes used outside hospitals and operated by carers to provide nutrition to patients who, for various reasons – such as being unable swallow or not fully conscious – require special measures of this kind.

peak flow meter: small plastic tube with a measuring indicator used to assess the strength of the outward breath. Useful for people with breathing problems, particularly people with asthma. These are available from health centres, although they can also be bought from chemists.

PEG (Percutaneous Endoscopic Gastrostomy): a thin tube inserted just under the skin directly into the stomach (a PEG feeding line). More recently PEG feeding is being replaced by a Radiologically Inserted Gastrostomy feeding tube (RIG).

pruritus: a symptom of other conditions, an uncomfortable sensation characterized by itchiness in various parts of the body – anus, vulva, skin – caused by irritation of a sensory nerve.

spirituality: the specific type of psychological care – often provided at the end of life – focusing on an evaluation of the person's values about life, whether linked to religious or non-religious belief.

terminal care: used to denote end-of-life care, when the person is at an advanced stage of their illness and is dying.

total pain: the physical, social, emotional, social, psychological and spiritual aspects of a person's well-being that influence the way they experience pain. The term was popularized by Cecily Saunders in the early 1960s.

toxic confusion (confusional state): confusion caused by toxins in the body often arising in older people due to a lack of fluids and seen when people are dehydrated (or uraemic) due to the build-up of urea in the body.

Index